OXFORD MEDIC⌐ .L PUI

CW00958655

Ne⸱   .cular Di

NEUROMUSCULAR DISEASES

JAAP BETHLEM
Professor of Neurology,
University of Amsterdam

and

CHARLOTTE E. KNOBBOUT
Physiotherapist
University of Amsterdam

OXFORD   NEW YORK   TOKYO
OXFORD UNIVERSITY PRESS
1987

Oxford University Press, Walton Street, Oxford OX2 6DP
Oxford New York Toronto
Delhi Bombay Calcutta Madras Karachi
Petaling Jaya Singapore Hong Kong Tokyo
Nairobi Dar es Salaam Cape Town
Melbourne Auckland
and associated companies in
Beirut Berlin Ibadan Nicosia

Oxford is a trade mark of Oxford University Press

Published in the United States
by Oxford University Press, New York

© Scheltema & Holkema, 1987

British Library Cataloguing in Publication Data
Bethlem, Jaap
Neuromuscular diseases.—(Oxford medical publications)
1. Neuromuscular diseases
I. Title   II. Knobbout, Charlotte E.
III. Neuromusculaire Ziekten. English
616.7'4   RC925.5
ISBN 0–19–261586–6

Library of Congress Cataloging-in-Publication Data
Bethlem, J.
Neuromuscular diseases.
(Oxford medical publications)
Translation of: Neuromusculaire ziekten.
Bibliography: p.
Includes index.
1. Neuromuscular diseases.   I. Knobbout, Charlotte E.
II. Title.   III. Series   [DNLM:
1. Neuromuscular Diseases—diagnosis.   WE 550 B562n]
RC925.5.B4713   1987   616.7'4   86-23590
ISBN 0–19–261586–6 (pbk.)

Set by Hope Services
Abingdon, Oxon
Printed in Great Britain by
The Alden Press, Oxford

Preface

There have been great advances in myology in recent decades, and it has gradually developed into a neurological subspecialty. Most medical workers have a limited knowledge of neuromuscular disease, however, and generally have to rely on specialist literature for any further information they require.

This book attempts to present a predominantly clinical and practical survey of the most important neuromuscular diseases. It has been written for everybody involved with patients suffering from these disorders, not only general practitioners, neurologists, paediatricians, rehabilitation specialists, and orthopaedic surgeons, but also physiotherapists and other exercise therapists, who are often intensively involved with patients for long periods of time. Thus, considerable attention is paid to the complaints presented by the patient and the signs that can be observed during physical examination. In addition, many chapters end with a PS, which can be read both as a postscript and as a 'provocative statement', with the aim of emphasizing certain practical problems and experiences.

Discussions with Dr Marianne de Visser, neurologist, who read through the entire manuscript several times, have been most valuable in the writing of this book. We are very grateful for her constant interest and constructive criticism.

Finally, we owe a special debt of gratitude to the many patients who kindly posed for the pictures and, in this way, helped to realize the aim of this book: to generate a better knowledge of neuromuscular diseases.

Amsterdam   J.B.
1986   Ch.E.K.

To Nelletje

Contents

He saw the hollow back, the thickened calves,
The cheerful child's problems getting to his feet.
The mother asked:
Will my son finish up in a wheelchair?
He, overcome with grief,
Decided not to share the truth with her . . .

1

Classification of neuromuscular diseases

A neurogenic disease is one in which muscle function is insufficient or absent owing to a primary disorder of the peripheral motor neuron (anterior horn cell, peripheral nerve). If muscle function is insufficient or absent because the muscle itself is diseased, a patient is said to have a myogenic disorder or myopathy. Disorders of the neuromuscular junction can also impair muscle function: myasthenia gravis is one of the best known examples.

All disorders of the peripheral motor neuron, the neuromuscular junction, and the muscle are called neuromuscular diseases (Table 1.1). There are several systems of classification, but the one that is used most often is that of the World Federation of Neurology. Table 1.2 represents a greatly abbreviated and modified version of this classification and an extensive list of neuromuscular diseases can be found in Walton's *Disorders of voluntary muscle* (1981).

Table 1.1 The neuromuscular diseases.

1 *Primary disorders of the peripheral motor neuron.*
   Diseases of the anterior horn cells (spinal muscular atrophies).
   Diseases of the peripheral nerves (neuropathies).

2 *Neuromuscular transmission disorders.*

3 *Primary disorders of the muscle.*
   (Myogenic diseases, or myopathies)

The problem in classifying neuromuscular diseases is that there is no firm basis from which to work. The causes of most of the disorders are unknown and for this reason an optimal classification (i.e., one based on aetiology) is not possible. Furthermore, both the classification and nomenclature of neuromuscular diseases have a historical base, with all its associated disadvantages.

1

Table 1.2 Classification of the neuromuscular diseases.

I *Disorders of the anterior horn cells.*
Proximal spinal muscular atrophies.
    Werdnig–Hoffmann disease.
      Wohlfart–Kugelberg–Welander disease.
Distal spinal muscular atrophy.
Scapuloperoneal spinal muscular atrophy.
Facioscapulohumeral spinal muscular atrophy.
Focal spinal amyotrophy.
Amyotrophic lateral sclerosis.
Infectious disorders.
    poliomyelitis anterior acuta.
Congenital and traumatic disorders.

II *Disorders of the peripheral nerves.*
Hereditary motor and sensory neuropathies.
Hereditary neuropathy with liability to pressure palsies.
Entrapment neuropathies.
Toxic neuropathies.
Metabolic neuropathies.
Neuropathies associated with infections.
Neuropathies associated with endocrine diseases.
Neuralgic amyotrophy.
Guillain–Barré syndrome.
Traumatic and toxic disorders.
Tumours of the peripheral nerves.

III *Neuromuscular transmission disorders.*
Myasthenia gravis.
Pseudocholinesterase deficiency.
Botulism.
Lambert–Eaton syndrome.

IV *Disorders of muscle.*
Genetically determined myopathies ('muscular dystrophies').
    Duchenne muscular dystrophy.
    Becker muscular dystrophy.
    facioscapulohumeral muscular dystrophy.
    scapuloperoneal syndrome.
    distal myopathies.
    ocular myopathies.
    oculopharyngeal myopathy.
Congenital myopathies.
    central core disease.
    multicore disease.

centronuclear myopathies.
nemaline myopathy.
Mitochondrial myopathies.
  morphologically abnormal mitochondria with known biochemical
    defect.
  morphologically abnormal mitochondria with unknown biochemical
    defect.
  morphologically normal mitochondria with known biochemical defect.
Myotonic disorders.
  myotonic dystrophy.
  myotonia congenita.
  chondrodystrophic myotonia.
  paramyotonia congenita.
Glycogen storage diseases.
  acid maltase deficiency.
  debranching enzyme deficiency.
  branching enzyme deficiency.
  muscle phosphorylase deficiency.
  phosphofructokinase deficiency.
Disorders of lipid metabolism in muscle.
  carnitine deficiencies.
  carnitine palmityltransferase deficiencies.
Periodic paralyses.
  familial hypokalaemic periodic paralysis.
  familial hyperkalaemic periodic paralysis.
  familial normokalaemic periodic paralysis.
  non-hereditary periodic paralyses.
Inflammatory myopathies.
  polymyositis.
  dermatomyositis.
  virus myositides.
  bacterial myositides.
  trichinosis.
  sarcoidosis.
  polymyalgia rheumatica.
Muscle disorders associated with endocrine diseases.
  thyrotoxic myopathy.
  hypothyroid myopathy.
  hyperparathyroid myopathy.
Other muscle disorders.
  paroxysmal myoglobinuria.
  malignant hyperthermia.
  disorders induced by medication, trauma, or toxins.
  tumours of the muscles.

The oldest classification refers to the so-called muscular dystrophies. This includes a group of diseases which have absolutely no relationship to each other. They were, and still are, classified on the basis of the most common site of muscle weakness (e.g., facioscapulophumeral dystrophy, ocular myopathy, distal myopathy, etc.). The 'myotonias' are classified as such if the sign myotonia is present. Diseases included in this group (e.g., myotonic dystrophy, myotonia congenita, and chondrodystrophic myotonia) have nothing else in common.

As for the large group of congenital myopathies, it appears that the main criterion for their classification is neither the site of muscle weakness nor any common sign, but rather the time at which the disorder became manifest (i.e., at birth).

A number of diseases that show similar morphologic features (e.g., the mitochondrial myopathies) have also been grouped together, despite the fact that the disorders themselves are hardly related to one another, if at all. The glycogen storage diseases associated with muscle weakness are classified in the best way; they are all based on a now known deficiency of one of the enzymes involved in glycogen metabolism.

Given the arbitrary nature of the classification, it is important to remember the relative value of the criteria used and, indeed, of the classification itself.

2

Genetics and neuromuscular diseases

Many neuromuscular diseases appear to be hereditary. In the case of autosomal dominant disease (Table 2.1), it is important to identify all heterozygotes (those suffering from the disease) since they can pass the disease to 50 per cent of their offspring. Most heterozygotes can be identified by the symptoms and signs present on examination.

Table 2.1 Autosomal dominant neuromuscular diseases.

Hereditary motor and sensory neuropathies.
Hereditary neuropathy with liability to pressure palsies.
Benign infantile spinal muscular atrophy (rare).
Facioscapulohumeral dystrophy.
Scapuloperoneal syndrome.
Ocular myopathy.
Oculopharyngeal myopathy.
Myopathia distalis tarda hereditaria.
Myotonic dystrophy.
Myotonia congenita (Thomsen).
Central core disease.
Nemaline myopathy.
Centronuclear myopathy.
Myotubular myopathy.
Multicore disease.
Periodic paralyses.
Muscle phosphorylase deficiency (rare).
Myopathies with abnormal mitochondria.
Malignant hyperthermia.

In many autosomal dominant neuromuscular diseases, however, the degree to which the gene is expressed varies and this may result in few clinical manifestations of the disease.

In facioscapulophumeral dystrophy, for example, the clinical picture can be limited to a weakness of the lower part of the facial muscles. The only complaint these patients have is that they can not whistle. It is clear that they will not consult a doctor because of this and will only mention it if specifically asked. In those suffering from myotonic dystrophy the myotonia may be very slight. In later life they may develop cataracts, but this alone will certainly not alert anyone to the fact that they have a 'muscular disease'.

It is as well to realize that such mildly affected patients may well have a child with a more serious form of the disease. It is known that mothers of children who have severe congenital myotonic dystrophy have a mild form of the disease themselves.

People are inclined to think that the disease has skipped a generation if they see that an adult, with a serious form of hereditary dominant muscular disease, has a child who has few complaints, if any, (although examination shows him to have the disease), and that child later has offspring in whom the disease is once again severe.

The way in which to recognize heterozygotes who show little sign of disease varies according to the neuromuscular condition. In the case of myotonic dystrophy, for example, a neurological examination combined with a slit-lamp examination is best. In hereditary neuropathy with liability to pressure palsies, or in hereditary motor and sensory neuropathies, however, it is important to determine the motor and sensory conduction velocities which occur in the peripheral nerves.

Heterozygotes with autosomal recessive diseases (Table 2.2), who show no clinical signs, can only pass the disorder to their offspring if their partner is also heterozygotic. They have a 25 per cent chance of having a child with the disease.

In practice, the heterozygotes of autosomal recessive neuromuscular diseases often go unrecognized, since they have no clinical signs of disease. This applies, for example, to the infantile spinal

Table 2.2 Autosomal recessive neuromuscular diseases.

Malignant infantile spinal muscular atrophy (Werdnig–Hoffmann disease).
Benign infantile, or juvenile, spinal muscular atrophy (Wohlfart–Kugelberg–Welander disease).
Juvenile progressive bulbar palsy (Fazio–Londe disease).
Hereditary motor and sensory neuropathies.
Scapuloperoneal syndrome.
Ocular myopathy.
Myotonia congenita (Becker).
Chondrodystrophic myotonia.
Central core disease.
Nemaline myopathy.
Centronuclear myopathy.
Myotubular myopathy.
Multicore disease.
Muscle phosphorylase deficiency.
Debranching enzyme deficiency.
Branching enzyme deficiency.
Phosphofructokinase deficiency.
Myopathies with abnormal mitochondria.

---

muscular atrophies (Werdnig–Hoffmann disease and Wohlfart–Kugelberg–Welander disease). If the healthy brothers or sisters of a patient with a recessive disorder ask whether they can pass the condition on to their offspring, they can be reassured that the chance of their doing so is so small as to be negligible, provided that the disorder does not occur in their partner's family and there is no consanguinity.

Those heterozygotes with acid maltase deficiency, can sometimes be recognized because they excrete less enzyme than normal in their urine or have less enzyme than normal in their muscle tissue or leucocytes. In the autosomal recessive form of nemaline myopathy, heterozygotes may be recognized through abnormalities of their muscle tissue (e.g., the presence of rods or central cores).

In X-linked recessive neuromuscular diseases (Table 2.3) the carrier of the gene has a 25 per cent chance of having an affected child and a 75 per cent chance of a healthy one or, to put it another way, a 50 per cent chance that her sons will suffer from this disease. Mentioning these percentages to the parent, however, may well lead to confusion in a genetic counselling session.

Table 2.3 X-linked recessive neuromuscular diseases.

Duchenne muscular dystrophy.
Becker-type muscular dystrophy.
Emery–Dreyfuss disease.
Scapuloperoneal syndrome.
Progressive proximal spinal and bulbar muscular atrophy (Kennedy).
'Myotubular' myopathy.
Mitochondrial myopathy with cardiomyopathy.

It is therefore recommended that risk percentages and other relevant information should be sent in writing to those seeking advice, after the consultation. Often a second consultation will prove necessary, especially if the 'bad news' appears to be poorly understood or hard to accept. Carriers of Duchenne muscular dystrophy can be identified by monitoring the activity of serum creatine kinase. However, no more than 80 per cent of carriers have an increase in CK activity. In Becker's disease only 50 per cent of carriers show an increase in serum creatine kinase. In this disease, however, the male patient reaches reproductive maturity, in contrast to the male with Duchenne muscular dystrophy, and all his daughters will be carriers. Carriers of 'myotubular' myopathy often have abnormal muscle tissue (small-diameter type 1 fibres, and sometimes small fibres resembling myotubules as well).

Genetic counselling is no easy matter, as none of the carriers of an X-linked recessive neuromuscular disease can be recognized with 100 per cent certainty. A great deal of experience and a thorough understanding of the problems involved are therefore of the utmost importance. For this reason, the genetic counselling of patients with neuromuscular disorders is best carried out by specialists in anthropogenetic institutes in conjunction with specialists in neuromuscular diseases.

3

Treatment of neuromuscular diseases

As shown in the previous chapter, many of the neuromuscular diseases are hereditary, which means that no effective treatment leading to recovery can ever be achieved. The best therapeutic results are often obtained with non-hereditary conditions such as myasthenia gravis and the polymyositis–dermatomyositis complex. In most neuromuscular diseases, symptomatic treatment, relying particularly on different forms of physiotherapy, can be of great importance to the patient. The prevention and treatment of contractures is often necessary, for example, in many neurogenic and myogenic diseases. In wheelchair patients serious pes equinus can be a hindrance when using the foot supports. Preventing flexion contractures of the hips and knees will not only make walking easier, but also aid lying down.

With serious pareses or paralyses of the legs (as, for example, in polyneuropathies and spinal muscular atrophies) symptoms often develop as a result of poor circulation in the lower legs and feet (cold feet, swollen feet, trophic abnormalities of the skin). These patients can also be helped by various types of physiotherapy (heat application, hot and cold baths, massage, passive movements) and advice (raising the feet when sitting or lying down). Many patients with neuromuscular disorders complain of pains which appear to be due to excessive use of the muscles and/or changes in posture. Here too, treatment aimed at a more efficient use of certain muscles or muscle groups, and postural instruction, can remove a lot of discomfort.

Very little scientific research has concentrated on the role of muscle-strengthening exercises in different neuromuscular diseases. It is not even known whether such exercises, particularly for patients with primary disorders of the muscle, have any use at all. In progressive diseases it is difficult to assess whether or not physiotherapy has influenced the course of the disease. On the other hand, it must be said that most patients find physiotherapy useful. The psychological effect of regular and intensive contact with the physiotherapist undoubtedly plays a role here. As not enough is known about the type of physiotherapy a patient with neuromuscular disease should undergo for optimal results, nor for how long they will need it, the topic will not be discussed further here. The whole field of rehabilitation and its associated problems, including the indications for artificial ventilation, also falls outside the scope of this book.

Drugs can give good results in some cases, for example, in myasthenia gravis, the polymyositis–dermatomyositis complex, periodic paralyses, and carnitine deficiencies. Drugs may also be considered for treating such complaints as muscle cramps and myotonia. Medication will be discussed in the relevant chapters.

The treatment of neuromuscular disease can also include prescribing a certain life-style. This is important in idiopathic rhabdomyolysis and carnitine palmityltransferase deficiency (preventing excessive muscle use), carnitine deficiency (avoiding long-term fasting), or in hereditary neuropathies with liability to pressure palsies (avoiding situations in which compression of a peripheral nerve could develop). Finally, the treatment of endocrine diseases associated with neuropathies or myopathies (hyper- and hypothyroidism, hyperparathyroidism, and diabetes mellitus) can also lead to complete recovery from the neuromuscular condition.

4

Testing muscle function

Inspection

Careful inspection of the patient suffering from a neuromuscular disease will provide much information about the location of the muscle weakness. (Fig. 4.1). After general examination of the patient it is best to be systematic and work upwards from the feet. A pelvic obliquity can often markedly affect the other findings of the inspection, and for that reason it can be useful to start with a determination of the position of the pelvis. When inspecting a patient with a neuromuscular disease, attention should be paid to the following:

Atrophy or (pseudo)hypertrophy of the muscles

It is important here to ask oneself whether there is real (pseudo)hypertrophy of a particular muscle or whether the muscle concerned only appears more developed because the other muscles are wasted. Thus, calf muscles may appear (pseudo)-hypertrophic because of a very marked atrophy of the upper leg muscles.

Changes in the normal curvature of the spinal column

On sagittal inspection it is useful to distinguish between an increased lumbar lordosis caused by a dorsal shift of the trunk and one due to the pelvis tilting forward. These two changes do not always occur at the same time. The patient will compensate for slight weakness of the m.gluteus maximus by shifting his trunk backwards in order to maintain his balance while standing.

In such a position there is an increased lumbar lordosis. If the weakness of the gluteus maximus increases, the pelvis will start to incline forward and this increases the lumbar lordosis even further (Fig. 4.2). The associated hip flexion can also be affected by the presence of shortened hip flexors.

A marked lumbar lordosis can also be caused by weakness of the abdominal muscles, but this occurs in only a minority of cases.

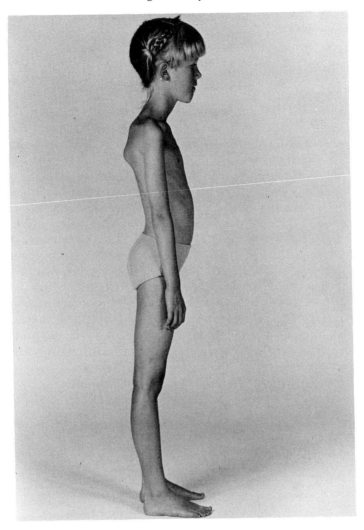

Fig. 4.1. Owing to the weakness of the gastrocnemius muscle, the ankle joint tends to plantar flexion. This weakness of the calf muscle together with the weakness of the quadriceps femoris muscle, gives rise to genu recurvatum. The marked lumbar lordosis is an indication of weakness of the extensors of the hip joint. There are also scapulae alatae due to weakness of the serratus anterior muscles. The head is held in anteposition to compensate for the lumbar lordosis.

Observation in the frontal plane will show up any scoliosis. An asymmetric weakening of the paravertebral musculature is possibly one of the causes of scoliosis in patients with neuromuscular disease. Scoliosis rarely occurs in patients with ambulatory-stage Duchenne muscular dystrophy. This can be explained by assuming that, as a result of the hyperlordotic posture during walking, the small lumbar facet joints move into a so-called close-packed position (or locking), which prevents a lateral deviation of the spinal column. If a scoliosis does occur in an ambulatory patient, there is usually a pelvic obliquity as a result of the contractures of the muscles around the pelvis and lower limbs.

A scoliosis will very often develop once the patient is confined to a wheelchair. One reason for this is that the spinal column is no longer maintained in sufficient extension to prevent a lateral collapse. Thus, by keeping the lumbar spine lordotic by means of a corset, one can attempt to prevent a scoliosis. In many patients with a thoracic scoliosis it has been observed that the convexity of the scoliosis points to the dominant limb. As a result of weakness in the muscles of the shoulder girdle, lateral flexion of the trunk towards the non-dominant side is required in order to be able to lift the shoulder of the dominant arm. This asymmetrically active force results in a scoliosis in which the convexity points towards the dominant limb.

Position of the legs and weight of the feet

Hyperextension of the knee joint (genu recurvatum) is observed when there is serious weakness of the m.quadriceps femoris and/or the m.gastrocnemius (see Fig. 4.1). A bilateral contracture of the m.tensor fasciae latae will not only further increase the forward tilt of the pelvis but will also increase the width of the base of support. If the patient does not put his weight on the entire foot, leaning mostly on the front part, there are two possibilities:
(1) There is a contracture of the m.gastrocnemius and the m.soleus.
(2) There is a weakness of the hip extensors and upper leg musculature combined with a contracture of the m.tensor fasciae latae.

The patient will stand on his toes to keep his balance (see p. 18).

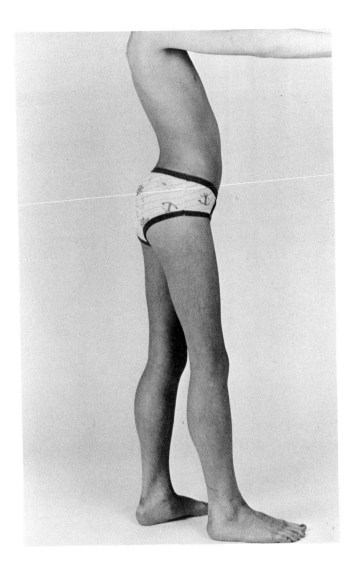

Fig. 4.2. A marked lumbar lordosis develops as a result of the weakness of the mm.glutei maximi. Both the dorsal shifting of the trunk and the forward tilting of the pelvis contribute to this lordosis. Hypertrophy of the calves can be noted as well.

Position of the shoulder girdle and arm

Medial rotation and 'winging' of the scapula (alata position) can be caused by a weakness of the m.serratus anterior (see Fig. 4.5) or by the rhomboideus (Fig. 4.3) and the pars transversus and pars

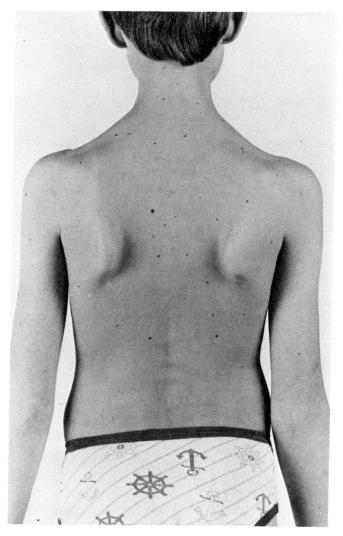

Fig. 4.3. In this patient the scapulae alatae proved to be caused by a weakness of the mm.rhomboidei rather than of the mm.serrati anteriores.

ascendens of the m.trapezius. If the back of the hand is turned forward instead of the thumb, a weakness of the medial rotators of the shoulder is indicated. A shortening of the m.pectoralis major may also give rise to lateral rotation of the arm. Contracture of the m.pectoralis minor is, as a rule, more likely to produce a shoulder protraction.

Facial expression

Weakness of the facial musculature may give rise to poor expression. This can be observed in, for example, myotonic dystrophy, facioscapulohumeral dystrophy, some congenital myopathies (see Table 17.2, p. 99), and myasthenia gravis. A severe bilateral ptosis is often compensated by contraction of the m.frontalis and/or retroflexion of the head.

A number of tests can be carried out after the inspection: *the Trendelenburg test* examines whether the m.gluteus medius and the m. gluteus minimus are strong enough to stabilize the pelvis with regard to the femur when standing on one leg. To carry out this test one stands behind the patient and asks him to raise his leg until hip and knee joints are held in 90 degree flexion. The test is considered to be positive if the pelvis descends on the side of the raised leg, indicating an insufficiency of the m. gluteus medius and/ or minimus of the leg the patient is standing on. The descent of only one side of the pelvis can often be seen better if the observer places both thumbs on the spinae iliacae posteriores and the other fingers horizontally on the cristae iliacae.

The test should always be carried out for both legs. Usually, if there is a severe weakness of the m.gluteus medius and minimus, the automatic compensation of the body is to move the centre of gravity over the hip by lateral trunk flexion towards the supported side. This phenomenon is called Duchenne's sign. A slight incline of the trunk will be directly visible if the observer holds his hands vertically under the patient's armpits. If the above phenomena occur during walking — tilting of the pelvis towards the unsupported side and lateral flexion of the trunk towards the supported side — this is called a Trendelenburg–Duchenne gait (see p. 18). *Gowers' sign* occurs with insufficiency of the m.gluteus maximus. The patient is asked to lie on his back on the floor and get up again. With a positive Gowers' sign the patient will carry out the following actions. First he turns on his side and then kneels, using his hands as support. Then he spreads his legs. Placing his hands flat on the floor in front of him, he puts his weight on them and, arms stretched, manœuvres himself into a position where his hips stick up in the air. From this forward-bending position, he places his hands on and above the knees and so climbs up his thighs, extending first the knees, then the hips and lastly the trunk, until he is standing erect (Fig. 4.4).

Testing the muscle power

Testing the muscle power of a patient with a neuromuscular disease does of course play an important role in the examination. There are a number of ways in which muscle power can be tested: functional testing, isolated manual testing and mechanical testing.

Functional testing of muscle power

Functional muscle testing involves observing the patient carry out a number of motor tests. It can be considered to supplement the inspection and the manual testing of muscles. The method has a number of advantages. Generally, the evaluation of these tests is relatively straightforward. For example: the patient is either able or unable to put his hands on his head. Subjective factors do not play such an important role here as in isolated manual testing.

The relatively simple tasks and the fact that they take so little time also make this type of test suitable for children. The less direct confrontation of the patient with any reduced muscle power can be viewed as a further advantage. Functional tests include: walking, standing or walking on one's heels, standing or walking on tiptoe, climbing on a chair, rising from a chair, standing up from a sitting position on the floor, and raising the arms.

Observation of gait. Research in this area has focused on children with Duchenne muscular dystrophy. A combination of progressive muscle weakness on the one hand, and the development of contractures on the other, means that the patients are no longer able to walk without support. In Duchenne muscular dystrophy the m.gluteus maximus is one of the first muscles to weaken. One of this muscle's functions is to stabilize the hip joint if the point of gravity lies forward of the hips when standing.

A patient with weakness of the m.gluteus maximus will bring the

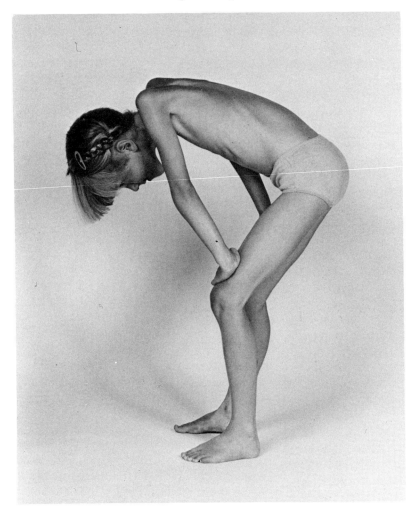

Fig. 4.4. Characteristic phase of Gowers' manœuvre: climbing up the legs to reach a standing position.

centre of gravity to the back of the hips to keep upright, using the iliofemoral ligamentum as a passive stabilizer. Shifting the point of gravity first becomes apparent as an increase in lumbar lordosis. Most of the fibres of the m.gluteus maximus radiate into the tractus iliotibialis. Weakness of the m.gluteus maximus will give the tractus a ventral position. Both the tractus iliotibialis and the m.tensor fasciae latae tend to become shorter in this position, which in turn increases hip flexion even more. At this point the patient has to increase the lumbar lordosis even further in order to keep his centre of gravity behind the hips. As the disease progresses, the m.quadriceps femoris may weaken further, thus posing a threat to the active stabilization of the knee. Passive stabilization of the knee can be achieved by bringing the centre of gravity in front of the knees, using the posterior part of the capsula and its attached ligaments. The patient must try to keep his weight behind the hips and in front of the knees, but, owing to the flexion contracture of the hips, the only way to achieve this is by walking on tiptoe. In this situation a fixed equinus position of the ankle is necessary to force the knee to extend. This position is, primarily, a compensatory mechanism for the insufficiency of the hip extensors and the upper leg musculature. In fact, the degree of contracture of the Achilles tendons is usually found to be relatively slight, which suggests there are other causes contributing to the equinus position.

The insufficiency of the m.gluteus medius and minimus poses a threat to lateral stability. To compensate, the patient adopts a Trendelenburg–Duchenne gait. As the muscle weakens further, walking becomes increasingly less safe. Finally, the patient walks on tiptoe, feet wide apart, and with a marked lordosis. When walking, the hip, knee, and ankle joints lie increasingly in a vertical line. To help keep the balance the arms are abducted and the neck bent forward, with the chin almost touching the chest.

Standing or walking on the heels. If the inability to stand or walk on the heels is due to an insufficiency of the foot dorsiflexors, compensation can be achieved by stretching the knees, pulling back the hips, and bringing the trunk slightly forward, thereby making it possible to lift the front of the feet. In many cases, however, the inability to stand or walk on the heels is not due to weakness of the foot dorsiflexors, but to a weakness of the hip extensors or upper leg musculature. This type of weakness actually forces the standing patient to bring his centre of gravity to the back of the hips and in front of the knees. With the balance being so precarious the patient would fall immediately if he stood on his heels.

In the case of severe weakness of the hip extensors and upper leg musculature, and with a flexion contracture of the hips, only standing on tiptoe will prevent a patient from losing his balance. In such cases, standing or walking on the heels is clearly impossible even with the function of the m.tibialis anterior fully intact. Patients with serious foot malformations (e.g. pes cavus) or changes in posture (e.g. pes equinus) are also unable to stand or walk on their heels.

Standing or walking on the toes. The inability to stand or walk on the toes is generally the result of weakness of the m.triceps surae.

Climbing on a chair. With a slight weakness of the hip extensors and upper leg musculature the patient will hesitate before stepping on a chair. One foot is placed on the chair and the patient clearly has to concentrate to place the other leg beside it. He bends the knee of the leg which is still on the ground, thus generating the thrust required to shift his weight to the leg on the chair. If there is more serious weakness of the pelvic girdle and upper leg musculature, the patient will fail to shift his weight forward sufficiently and will fall back on his rear leg. With an even more pronounced weakness he will no longer be able to place one leg on the chair. In these last two cases the patient may be asked to step on a low stool. Generally, a patient with severe weakness will only manage to do this if he can hold on to something near the low stool. With one foot on the stool he will place a hand on his knee and thus help stretch his knee during the step up. Similarly, the trunk is brought forward quickly to aid the push up. The patient must be instructed to carry out this test using each leg in turn. By leaving it up to the patient which leg to use first, information can be obtained as to which leg is best (preferred leg).

Rising from a chair. When there is weakness of the hip extensors, the patient will use one or both hands on the arm rests to push himself up. If there is an additional weakness of the knee extensors the patient will subsequently put his hands on his knees. The knees are then stretched with the aid of the hands. The patient is now bending forwards. By 'climbing up' his legs with his hands he is able to stand upright again.

Standing up from sitting on the floor. Weakness of the m.gluteus maximus gives rise to Gowers' sign (see p. 16).

Elevation of the arms. If a patient with weakness of the m.deltoideus and the m.supraspinatus, raises and abducts his arms one may observe a compensatory contraction of the m.trapezius

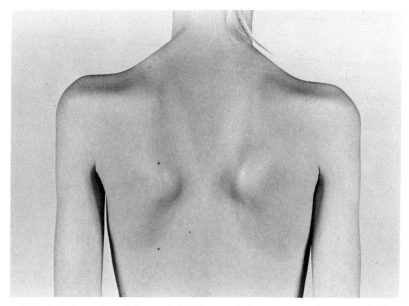

Fig. 4.5. Atrophy of the m.deltoideus and the m.supraspinatus on both sides. There are also scapulae alatae as a result of weakness of the mm.serrati anteriores.

much earlier than normal. In the case of scapulae alatae, the fixation of the shoulder blade which is necessary to achieve arm abduction, may be insufficient to the extent that abduction is no longer possible. If, however, the examiner immobilizes the shoulder blade then it is possible to carry out this movement provided the m.deltoideus and the m.supraspinatus are both intact. This situation occurs frequently in facioscapulohumeral dystrophy (see p. 78). During elevation with anteflexion the use of the trunk to 'throw up' the arms can also point to a weakness in the shoulder girdle musculature. This manœuvre can often be seen when shaking the patient's hand.

If the patient is requested to keep his arms in a 90 degree anteflexion position, a compensatory increase in contraction of the m.trapezius descendens will take place (Fig. 4.5 and 4.6).

If the weakness of the shoulder-girdle musculature develops further the patient will no longer be able to lift his arms above his head. In this case one should note just how high the patient can lift

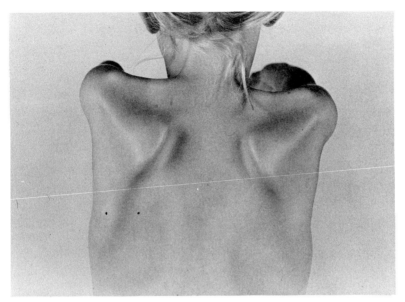

Fig. 4.6. There is increased winging of the scapulae during elevation with anteflexion of the arms. The trapezius descendens muscles compensate by contracting excessively.

them. The way the patient takes off a sweater will also provide clues about the condition of the shoulder-girdle and arm musculature. If there is severe weakness of the shoulder-girdle musculature, he will place his elbows on the table and then bend forward to pull the sweater over his head with his hands.

Other arm-function tests. In the case of distally located weakness, the patient has difficulty in carrying an object (e.g. a shopping bag). In time he may no longer be able to undo buttons, unscrew lids or engage in other activities requiring the power of the small hand muscles. Such activities can also be used as test assignments.

Manual testing of individual muscles

The most often used classification here is that of the Medical Research Council. The MRC scale, as it is called, dates from 1943 (Table 4.1). In practice, it is soon obvious that the six grades on the MRC scale are often insufficient to describe the findings, and

Table 4.1 Classification of muscle power according
to the Medical Research Council (MRC scale).

Grade 0. No contraction.
Grade 1. Flicker or trace of contraction.
Grade 2. Active movement with gravity eliminated.
Grade 3. Active movement against gravity.
Grade 4. Active movement against gravity and resistance.
Grade 5. Normal power.

for that reason these grades are often elaborated with minuses and pluses. These additions, however, do not as a rule give any more accurate classification of the degree of weakness. Everybody who has tested muscle power using the MRC scale, has experienced that colleagues apply this refinement of adding plus or minus signs in a different way. Another disadvantage is that some muscles e.g., the m.rhomboideus or the m.latissimus dorsi, cannot be tested fully against gravity.

It is necessary to be systematic when testing muscle power. Thus, it is important to record whether the examiner tests the power during a concentric isometric (static) or during an eccentric contraction of the muscle. If, for example, the m.quadriceps femoris needs to be tested, the patient is asked to sit on the edge of the examination bench, his knees bent. If the examiner gives resistance to the front of the lower leg while the patient attempts to extend his knee, a contraction of the m.quadriceps femoris (concentric contraction) will follow. Thus, the turning moment of the muscle exceeds that of the opposing forces.

An isometric contraction of the m.quadriceps femoris takes place if the examiner fixes the leg in a 180 degree extension of the knee joint and asks the patient to maintain this position against pressure. The word isometric (equal length) is in fact wrongly applied to this situation because there will always be some change in length, however small. For that reason the term static contraction is sometimes used as well. This refers to the fact that the turning moment of the muscle equals the turning moment of the opposing forces.

If the examiner provides enough resistance to bend the 180-degree-stretched leg, then an eccentric contraction of the

Table 4.2 Grading of functional abilities

According to Swinyard, Deaver, and Greenspan (1957).

(1) Ambulates with waddling gait and marked lordosis. Elevation activities adequate (climbs stairs and kerbs without assistance).

(2) Ambulates with waddling gait and marked lordosis. Elevation activities deficient (needs support for kerbs and stairs).

(3) Ambulates with waddling gait and marked lordosis. Cannot negotiate kerbs or stairs, but can achieve erect posture from a standard height chair.

(4) Ambulates with waddling gait and marked lordosis. Unable to rise from a standard height chair.

(5) Wheelchair independence; good posture in the chair; can perform all activities of daily living from chair.

(6) Wheelchair with dependence: can roll chair, but needs assistance in bed and wheelchair activities.

(7) Wheelchair with dependence and back support. Can roll the chair only a short distance, needs back support for good chair position.

(8) Bed patient: can do no activities of daily living without maximum assistance.

According to Vignos, Spencer, and Archibald (1963).

(1) Walks and climbs stairs without assistance.

(2) Walks and climbs stairs with aid of railing.

(3) Walks and climbs stairs slowly with aid of railing (over 25 seconds for eight standard steps).

(4) Walks unassisted and rises from chair, but cannot climb stairs.

(5) Walks unassisted, but cannot rise from chair or climb stairs.

(6) Walks only with assistance or walks independently with long leg braces.

(7) Walks in long leg braces, but requires assistance for balance.

(8) Stands in long leg braces, but unable to walk even with assistance.

(9) Is in wheelchair. Can flex elbows against gravity.

(10) Is in wheelchair or bed. Cannot flex elbows against gravity.

---

m.quadriceps femoris takes place. During contraction the muscle lengthens, making the muscle turning moment less than that of the opposing forces.

Generally, it appears that a muscle uses less energy for an eccentric contraction than for a concentric. In other words, a larger force can be developed with an eccentric contraction than with a concentric or static contraction using the same load.

This can be observed, for example, in a patient with weakness of the m.deltoideus. This patient is no longer able to abduct his arm against gravity (concentric contraction). However, if the examiner places the arm in a 90 degree abduction position, it does not fall back immediately against the body, but sinks down gradually as a result of the eccentric contraction of the m.deltoideus. The book *Muscles*, by Kendall, Kendall, and Wadsworth (1971) gives an excellent survey of the testing of muscle function and power. However, whether or not muscles can be tested individually remains an open question.

Mechanical testing of muscle power

Measuring muscle power by means of dynamometers or other measuring equipment is still mostly at an experimental stage. The application of mechanical tests in patients with a neuromuscular disease often appears to be difficult. The large number of paretic muscles, the resulting difficulties with fixations no longer taking place normally, and the possible influence that contractures may exert on the test situation itself, all contribute to the fact that it is often impossible to test muscle power by such mechanical means.

Apart from recording muscle power, it is equally important, especially for rehabilitation purposes, to assess the patient's motor skills. Several classifications have been developed for this purpose; two which are often used are presented in Table 4.2. Finally, normal psychomotor development must also be taken into account when evaluating muscle tests in children.

5

Spinal muscular atrophies

The spinal muscular atrophies form a group of neuromuscular diseases in which the primary lesion is located in the anterior horn cells of the spinal cord. In some of these diseases there is also involvement of the cranial nerves (Table 5.1). For reasons unknown the anterior horn cells degenerate, giving rise to clinical signs such as paresis or paralysis, muscular atrophy, fasciculation and areflexia. The autosomal recessive, proximal spinal muscular atrophies are most frequent; the distal and scapuloperoneal forms are much less so, and other types are rare.

Infantile spinal muscular atrophy
(Werdnig–Hoffmann disease)

This is an autosomal recessive disorder and 30 per cent of mothers notice, during pregnancy, that their unborn babies are less active. In 95 per cent of the patients the signs become manifest before the fourth month, while only a few months later signs of motor retardation can be observed in all patients. The syndrome of arthrogryposis multiplex congenita can sometimes occur immediately after birth. Most of the children, however, are floppy infants with generalized hypotonia and muscle weakness. Initially, the weakness is more pronounced in the muscles of the pelvic girdle and legs than in the shoulder-girdle and arm musculature, while, in the limbs, the proximal muscle groups are more affected than the distal. In the course of a few months, however, the muscle weakness spreads and almost all muscle groups are equally affected. Once put in their cots, children will remain lying in the same position because the weakness of their muscles does not allow them to turn over or raise their head. The weakness of the intercostal muscles gives rise to respiratory disorders, while the bulbar muscles may become involved as well, leading to difficulties in feeding.

Although atrophy of the muscles is present, this is often masked by the layer of subcutaneous fat. For the same reason it is often

25

Table 5.1 Spinal muscular atrophies.

Proximal spinal muscular atrophy.	
Infantile spinal muscular atrophy (Werdnig–Hoffmann disease).	Autosomal recessive.
Intermediate spinal muscular atrophy (Fried–Emery).	Autosomal recessive.
Chronic infantile or juvenile spinal muscular atrophy (Wohlfart–Kugelberg–Welander disease).	Autosomal recessive.
Chronic proximal spinal muscular atrophy.	Autosomal dominant.
Progressive proximal spinal and bulbar muscular atrophy (Kennedy).	X-linked recessive.
Distal spinal muscular atrophy.	Autosomal recessive. Autosomal dominant.
Juvenile type of distal and segmental muscular atrophy of upper extremities.	Sporadic
Focal spinal amyotrophy.	Sporadic.
Scapuloperoneal spinal muscular atrophy.	Autosomal dominant. X-linked recessive. Sporadic.
Facioscapulohumeral spinal muscular atrophy.	Autosomal dominant. Sporadic.
Progressive juvenile bulbar palsy (Fazio–Londe disease).	Autosomal recessive.

impossible to observe fasciculations. Atrophy and fibrillations, however, can be seen in the tongue.

The reflexes are absent. Serum creatine kinase activity is almost always normal. Understandably, it is not always possible to carry out an electromyography on an infant, but the presence of fibrillations and spontaneous positive denervation potentials can contribute to the diagnosis.

Given the seriousness of the condition and its poor prognosis, in addition to the fact that many diseases can show the floppy-infant syndrome, it is important to confirm the diagnosis by muscle biopsy. The biopsy presents a very typical picture. There are two muscle fibre populations: normal (or hypertrophic) fibres which usually show the enzyme-histochemical properties of type-1 fibres, and small fibres, as well as a round shape in transverse section. Sometimes the fasciculi consist of small fibres only; sometimes there are only a few normal fibres scattered among the small fibres. One has the impression that the fibres have not become atrophic but that the small fibres were abnormally small from the start. If so it may well be more accurate to call the muscle fibres hypotrophic rather than atrophic. Changes in structure, particularly target fibres, are extremely rare.

The prognosis of Werdnig–Hoffmann disease is poor. Approximately 95 per cent of the children die, before they are 18 months old, of respiratory-tract infections caused by food aspiration and progressive breathing difficulties. Children rarely live beyond 4 years of age and those who do never learn to walk.

Intermediate form of infantile spinal muscular atrophy

This form usually commences between the third and eighteenth month. Initially, motor development may be normal and the progression less rapid than in Werdnig–Hoffmann disease. However, fewer than 25 per cent of the children can sit up straight without support, crawling is rarely achieved, and walking never. Sometimes the reflexes are there at the beginning, but by the time the child is 2 years old, they have generally disappeared. Not all authors assume that a separate intermediate form exists. They think that there is a gradual transition from Werdnig–Hoffmann disease to Wohlfart–Kugelberg–Welander disease. These authors are inclined to assume that Werdnig–Hoffmann disease and Wohlfart–Kugelberg–Welander disease are different expressions of the same condition.

Chronic infantile or juvenile spinal muscular atrophy (Wohlfart–Kugelberg–Welander disease)

This autosomal recessive disease occurs frequently, but there are no reliable data regarding its prevalence and incidence. The age of onset varies considerably, ranging from the first years of life to the thirties. Muscular weakness always begins in the upper legs and pelvic girdle. The first symptoms are a difficulty in climbing stairs, a waddling gait, inability to run, and falling down frequently and not being able to get up without support. Over several years the muscle weakness will spread to the shoulder girdle and upper arm muscles. In this way the picture of a limb-girdle syndrome builds up. It is therefore generally assumed that many of these patients were previously diagnosed as having limb-girdle muscular dystrophy. The neck muscles and the distal musculature eventually become involved in the process. In approximately 25 per cent of the patients, bulbar muscles (facial muscles, tongue) will weaken as well, although signs of bulbar palsy do not predominate in the clinical picture.

Atrophy of the weakened muscles occurs at an early stage. According to some authors varying degrees of hypertrophy of the calf muscles occur as well, possibly to compensate for the weakness of the dorsiflexors of the feet and toes. Fasciculations occur predominantly in the tongue, shoulder girdle, and upper arm muscles. However, these are only observed in just over 30 per cent of patients. Tremor of the fingers is also seen in approximately 30 per cent of cases. The presence of fasciculations and tremor of the fingers in patients with a limb-girdle syndrome strongly suggests a diagnosis of spinal muscular atrophy. The reflexes are usually absent, particularly in the lower limbs. A general areflexia is observed in half the patients; it is rare for all reflexes to be present. Babinski's reflex may occur in 1–3 per cent of the patients. Therefore, the presence of extensor plantar reflexes alone does not contradict this diagnosis, but, in such cases, it is advisable to bear in mind the possibility of an alternative diagnosis.

As a rule, serum creatine kinase activity is slightly to moderately increased. In children creatine kinase activity may be normal, increasing gradually during puberty. In fact, there is no constant correlation between serum creatine kinase and age, duration, or severity of the illness. The electromyogram shows signs of denervation (spontaneous fibrillation potentials and positive sharp waves, as well as long duration, high amplitude motor unit potentials), but short duration, low amplitude polyphasic action potentials can be observed as well. The conduction velocities of the motor and sensory nerves are normal.

Computed tomography of the skeletal musculature reveals low-density foci diffused over the entire muscle. The most extensive abnormalities are found in the muscles of the upper leg, and all muscles appear to be affected. Muscle biopsy will show the kind of alterations consistent with a peripheral motor neuron disorder: groups of small-diameter fibres with either an angular or a round shape in transverse sections. Sometimes, enzyme-histochemistry also shows a predominance of type-I or type-II fibres in addition to type-grouping.

The speed of progression can vary widely. Of great practical importance is the fact that bed rest (for example, during an infectious disease or after a small orthopaedic operation such as lengthening of the Achilles tendon) has an adverse effect on the course of the disease. Many patients report that walking becomes worse after a period of immobilization. Sometimes they even report that the first signs of the disease occurred after confinement to bed.

The life expectancy of patients who have never walked is lower than that of those who once were able to walk. If children do not make clear attempts at standing or walking by the time they are 5 years old, they are unlikely ever to do so. If the signs are clearly present in infants under 1 year of age, then there is a considerable chance they will end up in a wheelchair before the age of 20. However, there are also patients in whom the disease becomes manifest later in life; here the progression is so slow that a patient may remain able to walk for many decades.

As the disease progresses and more muscles become weak or paralytic, the danger of contractures and/or a (torsion) scoliosis grows; this is sometimes associated with thorax malformations. Flexion contractures of the hip and knee joints occur frequently, but foot deformations (pedes equinovari, talipes, flat feet, pedes equinovalgi and their various combinations) can also be observed at an early stage of the disease. Naturally, physiotherapy can be useful in keeping the patient mobile, but surgery (e.g. lengthening the Achilles tendon in pes equinus contractures) should be postponed as long as possible. The beneficial results for patients are not only rare, but the ability to walk usually deteriorates too, owing to the necessary post-operative bed rest or immobilization.

With physiotherapy, one must bear in mind that the exercise tolerance of the patients has often decreased and that they may develop cramps immediately after muscular exercise.

X-linked progressive proximal spinal and bulbar muscular atrophy

The first signs become apparent between the ages of 30 and 50 and usually consist of muscle cramps and fasciculations. These latter can precede by years a weakness and atrophy of the proximal muscles — usually of the legs — the tongue and the m.orbicularis oris. At a later stage the distal muscle groups may become involved and a relatively mild dysphagia and dysarthria may develop as well. There is often a tremor of the fingers. The reflexes are decreased or absent. There are never any signs of upper motor neuron involvement. The sensory system is also intact. The progression of the disease is very slow and may last many years, the patients attaining old age. The frequent occurrence of gynaecomastia is remarkable and remains unexplained. Recently, a growing number of studies of this disease have appeared; the disease probably occurs more often than was earlier assumed.

Distal spinal muscular atrophy

This is a relatively rare condition with onset at any age, although it usually begins between 10 and 20 years of age. The disease generally manifests itself in the form of foot deformations (pes cavus) and difficulties in walking as a result of weakness of the extensors of the feet and toes. An additional weakness and wasting of the lower arms and small muscles of the hands in a later stage only occurs in about 25 per cent of the patients. It is rare for the disease to commence with weakness and wasting of the small muscles of the hands. Some patients have a history of muscle cramps in their lower legs. Fasciculations are repeatedly reported or are observed during the examination.

Although ankle jerks are generally absent, other reflexes remain.

It is particularly important to differentiate the disease from the common hereditary motor and sensory neuropathies (see p. 48). Sensory disorders, however, are never found in distal spinal muscular atrophy and the motor and sensory conduction velocities are normal.

Juvenile distal and segmental muscular atrophy of the upper extremities

This has been described among Japanese and other Asians, but it is also observed in the West. Onset is usually between the ages of 18 and 22, and men are five times more likely to be affected than women. The patients first complain of fatigue in their fingers and a difficulty with the fine finger movements of one hand. Sometimes the muscle weakness only becomes manifest in cold weather (cold paresis). Gradually, atrophy and weakness of the lower arm and small muscles of the hand develop, as well as fasciculations. Weakness of the upper arm (m.triceps) and sensory defects may occur in about 20 per cent of patients. Very characteristic of the disease is the fact that the process is often unilateral and can become bilateral in one-third of the patients; it is always restricted to the upper limbs and there is no further progression after a few years. The condition often affects men who were accustomed to heavy muscular exercise or who were active sportsmen. In some patients computed tomography reveals a central cavity in the cervical part of the spinal cord.

Focal spinal amyotrophy

Focal spinal amyotrophy, also called benign focal amyotrophy, monomelic amyotrophy, or wasted-leg syndrome is a rather rare form of spinal muscular atrophy. Muscular atrophy and weakness are either strictly unilateral or asymmetrical. The condition has an insidious onset and shows very slow progression, if any. Men are mainly affected. There is a marked variation in the age of onset and in the distribution of weakness and atrophy.

Scapuloperoneal spinal muscular atrophy

In this rare form of spinal muscular atrophy the muscle weakness and atrophy is initially limited to the shoulder-girdle muscles and the extensors of the feet and toes. Progression is slow and the muscles of the pelvic girdle and upper legs weaken very gradually.

This condition should be distinguished from the scapuloperoneal myopathies (see p. 83). However, this is not always easy and may be impossible on the basis of electromyography and histopathology of a muscle biopsy. On the one hand the evaluation of a biopsy from the highly atrophic scapuloperoneal muscles, which have often been affected for a long time, is often not feasible because most of the muscle tissue has been replaced by fatty and connective tissue. On the other hand, a biopsy from a clinically unaffected muscle will often show either a normal picture or such slight and aspecific changes that no diagnosis can be made. It is particularly difficult to establish whether there is a primary neurogenic or myogenic lesion. The same holds true, *mutatis mutandis*, for electromyographic investigations. Besides, although the occurrence of brief, low-voltage, polyphasic action potentials suggests a myogenic disorder, it does not exclude the presence of a chronic neurogenic lesion.

Facioscapulohumeral spinal muscular atrophy

This rare disease is more common in later life, the weakness being limited to the muscles of the face, shoulders and upper arms. The condition must be distinguished from facioscapulohumeral dystrophy (Landouzy–Déjérine disease, see p. 77). Neurogenic abnormalities in the muscle biopsy are also observed in this latter disease which often makes it extremely difficult to establish the diagnosis with certainty.

Juvenile progressive bulbar palsy (Fazio–Londe disease)

This is a rare autosomal recessive condition; the disease begins in childhood with weakness — often unilateral — of the facial muscles, followed by difficulties in swallowing. Gradually bulbar paresis develops, sometimes with involvement of the extraocular muscles as well. Weakness of the musculature of the limbs may develop at a later stage.

Postscript

The most frequent cause of the limb-girdle syndrome is benign infantile spinal muscular atrophy or Wohlfart–Kugelberg–Welander disease.

A slight to moderate increase in serum creatine kinase does not contradict the diagnosis of Wohlfart–Kugelberg–Welander disease.

Patients with Wohlfart–Kugelberg–Welander disease must choose a job which they can continue to do as their disability progresses.

Try to keep patients with Wohlfart–Kugelberg–Welander disease as mobile as possible. This means, amongst other things, staying in bed as briefly as possible during any intervening illness, and postponing orthopaedic operations for as long as possible.

Keeping orthopaedic aids in the cupboard does not reflect well on the doctor involved.

Malignant infantile spinal muscular atrophy or Werdnig–Hoffmann disease is autosomal recessive. Parents of a child with this fatal disease should be informed of this (even if they themselves have not asked for any genetic advice).

6

Amyotrophic lateral sclerosis

Amyotrophic lateral sclerosis (ALS) is a disease in which, for reasons unknown, all the motor cells begin to degenerate. The clinical signs involved are therefore based as much on upper as on lower motor neuron involvement. The incidence varies from approximately 0.5–1.8 per 100 000 people (it is much higher on the island of Guam and on the Kii peninsula of Japan). The disease appears to be hereditary in about 5 per cent of cases; the autosomal dominant form being most common. It is more likely to be seen in men than in women, with a sex ratio between 1.5:1 and 1.8:1.

The condition occurs, as a rule, between the ages of 40 and 50 years, although it may occur at any time in adults. In general, the patients die 3 years after their first signs appear. Sometimes their life expectancy is shorter (e.g. in patients who developed a bulbar paralysis at an early stage). The disease rarely lasts longer than 5 years, especially in younger patients in whom the only clinical signs concern the anterior horn motor cells. Previously, this form of ALS was called progressive spinal muscular atrophy (Duchenne–Aran disease). There are still authors who consider this form to be a separate disease with a far more benign course than ALS.

The initial symptoms and signs consist of muscle cramps and/or fasciculations. If asked, 40 per cent of patients will complain of rapidly developing and often painful muscle cramps, especially after certain movements. Often the cramps will occur at night impairing sleep. They may precede the motor disorder by months or even years. As the disease progresses, the cramps diminish and eventually disappear altogether.

There is wide variety as regards the first signs of muscular weakness. For this reason, the correct diagnosis is often missed in the initial stage of the disease. The further course of the disease is also erratic and difficult to predict, and one is well advised to take this into account in the way the patient is approached. In more than half the patients, the first signs of muscle weakness occur in one arm only, namely in the small muscles of the hand (thenar eminence, m.interosseus primus). As a result the patient will experience difficulty with small movements of the fingers, for example, when doing up buttons or writing. This muscle weakness will be accompanied by wasting from an early stage. In classical cases the weakness will extend proximally, first to the flexors and then to the extensors of the fingers, the m.biceps, the m.triceps, the m.deltoideus and the other muscles of the shoulder girdle. Simultaneously, or soon afterwards, these abnormalities will also appear in the other hand and arm. Since the course of the disease is so varied and erratic one must bear in mind that muscle weakness and wasting may also begin in the shoulder muscles, leaving the distal musculature relatively unaffected for a long time.

The long muscles of the back, and the m.serratus anterior and the m.pectoralis major, may become involved in this process at an early stage. Neck muscles are affected far less often. Later, the pelvic and leg muscles weaken and waste, again asymmetrically at first. Finally, signs develop which point to involvement of the motor nuclei of the brain-stem. Such a bulbar paralysis will often commence with unilateral atrophy of the tongue and fasciculations. The latter are best observed if the patient is asked to open his mouth and flatten his tongue. As the process develops, dysphagia, dysarthria and difficulty in mastication will occur. Both upper and lower motor neurons are involved. Consequently, pseudobulbar reflexes (snout-reflex, compulsive crying, compulsive laughing, and a markedly brisk masseter reflex) occur repeatedly. Solids will often get stuck at the back of the throat when swallowing. Drinking often leads to choking, and the fluid will frequently be expelled through the nose. The saliva is not swallowed either; it accumulates in the pharynx where it provokes coughing and a feeling of choking. Speech impairment may lead to complete anarthria, when all the patient can produce, with difficulty, is a kind of growling.

The final phase of ALS is agonizing both for the patient and those close to him. Whereas consciousness remains intact until the end, as do sight and hearing, the patient is no longer able to move his arms and legs. Breathing is hampered, swallowing becomes almost impossible and the patient often feels as if he is choking on his saliva. As he can no longer speak, his only means of communicating with the world outside is by moving his eyes.

ALS begins with weakening and wasting of the dorsal flexors of the foot in about 25 per cent of patients. After some weeks or months the other leg will weaken as well so that the patient walks with a footdrop in both feet. As the ankle and sometimes the knee jerks may also be absent at this stage, polyneuropathy is often diagnosed. This form of ALS is also called the lumbar, peroneal or pseudo-polyneuropathic type. The absence of sensory impairment, the presence of fasciculations in both affected and unaffected muscles, and observation of the further course of the disease can eventually lead to the correct diagnosis.

Finally, a bulbar type is also distinguished in approximately 25 per cent of patients; in this form the disease first manifests itself in weakness of the bulbar musculature. Eventually the muscles of the arms, trunk and legs will become involved as well. The signs of an upper motor neuron lesion may be very slight or unapparent for some considerable time. Very brisk reflexes are often the only sign of involvement of the pyramidal tracts. The combination of weakness and wasting of the small muscles of the hands and forearms with very brisk arm reflexes strongly suggests a diagnosis of ALS, especially if fasciculations are present as well. Although the finger-snapping reflex and continuous ankle and patellar clonus are not rare, many patients do not show extensor plantar reflexes and other pathological reflexes of the foot, while the abdominal reflexes remain intact for a long time.

As mentioned before, fasciculations occur very early in the disease process without any apparent muscle weakness or atrophy. Later, fasciculations are observed not only in the paretic muscles but also in the non-paretic, and they continue during sleep. The presence of fasciculations provides an important clinical contribution to the diagnosis. It is of great importance, therefore, to establish whether they are present. This is not difficult in most patients since fasciculations are present in numerous muscles. Sometimes the fasciculations are so massive that they produce myoclonus-like movements. There are patients, however, in whom fasciculations can only be established with great difficulty. Twitching can be seen to increase if the patient is in cold surroundings, but this is of little practical use for a doctor who examines his patient in a heated examination room. What is important is that fasciculations occur for a short time after several strong contractions of the muscle involved. Percussion of the muscle with a percussion hammer will often provoke fasciculations as well.

Although patients may complain of paresthesias in the hands, feet or other parts of the body, disturbances of sensation are not part of the clinical picture. Although there are several publications which report signs of sensory dysfunction and neuropathological changes in the posterior columns, it is nevertheless good clinical practice, in the first instance, to reject the diagnosis of ALS if sensory abnormalities are present. The sensory evoked responses and nerve conduction velocities are also always normal. A remarkably large number of patients complain of pain as the disease progresses often the result of stiff joints, especially shoulder joints. If the patient is no longer able to turn over, he can suffer pain as a result of skin pressure as well. The motor nerve conduction velocities, on the other hand, may be reduced to low-normal or abnormal, especially if the muscles involved are very wasted. In this context special attention should be paid to the temperature of the limb. In healthy people a decrease in temperature results in a lower motor conduction velocity. The temperature of a very wasted and almost paralytic limb is often quite a lot lower in ALS patients, and for that reason it also has an effect on conduction velocity. As a general rule the conduction velocities of the motor and sensory nerves are normal, but a lowered motor conduction velocity does not argue against the diagnosis of ALS. This is of particular practical importance in the pseudopolyneuropathic form.

Electromyography is important, especially in the early stages of the disease, to demonstrate that the anterior horn cells are affected at different levels of the spinal cord. In this way neurogenic abnormalities can be demonstrated in clinically normal muscles as well. Neurogenic abnormalities in the EMG of the legs suggests ALS rather than cervical myelopathy. A muscle biopsy can also demonstrate neurogenic abnormalities in an otherwise healthy muscle. For that matter, histopathological findings in the muscle biopsy are the same as for any other lower motor neuron disorder. Thus it is impossible for a muscle biopsy to distinguish whether the primary lesion is in the anterior horn cells or in the peripheral nerve. As a rule, however, it is possible to discover the site of the primary lesion by neurophysiological examination.

Consequently, when diagnosing ALS, careful clinical examination and electromyography are far more important than the histopathological examination of a muscle biopsy.

In about half the patients, there is a slight increase in protein in the cerebrospinal fluid and a two- to threefold increase in serum creatine kinase activity.

As ALS is a fatal disease, feelings of fear, uncertainty and powerlessness on the part of the doctor in charge are often the reason why he tends to invite his patient for a check-up less and less often. During the check-up the patient is given a very superficial examination, if at all, and then sent home with the advice to come back 'if there are any complaints'. From his side, progressive disablement, with its reduction in mobility, and the realization that 'there is not a thing that the doctor can do' cause the patient to stop seeking medical help. Thus, it is often the physiotherapist with whom the patient remains in contact and from whom he receives support. Yet intensive medical support of both the patient and his family remains vital. An individually tailored rehabilitation programme may noticeably improve the patient's condition. Exercise therapy, breathing exercises, regular tapotement and aspiration of mucus from the pharynx, orthopaedic aids and special adaptations to the home are important in this context. Dietary measures should often be taken as well, particularly when the patient has difficulty in swallowing solids. When there is serious difficulty in swallowing, a cricopharyngeal myotomy must be considered. There is no known drug which stops the progressive degeneration of motor cells.

Postscript

Muscle cramps after muscle exercise or certain movements are usually the first complaint in ALS. They also occur at night and can be very painful.

Similarly, fasciculations are often the first sign of ALS. They can be provoked by strong repetitive muscle contractions and percussion of the muscle and may often be observed in clinically healthy muscles.

Clinical examination is the ideal method of diagnosing ALS.

Electromyography is especially important in the demonstration of neurogenic abnormalities at different levels of the spinal cord. These abnormalities can also be found in clinically non-paretic muscles.

A muscle biopsy is not always indicated and, in any case, does not provide evidence of whether the primary lesion is located in the anterior horn cells or the peripheral nerves.

The combination of weakness and wasting of small muscles of the hand and the forearm, fasciculations and noticeably brisk arm reflexes are strongly suggestive of ALS.

No diagnostic test is known to substantiate an ALS diagnosis.

7

Neuropathies

The neuropathies include a very large group of divergent disorders of the peripheral nerves with an acute, subacute or chronic course. The condition can manifest itself as a polyneuropathy, with the distal parts of the limbs being affected symmetrically. As a rule, the feet and lower legs are affected more than the hands and forearms. Usually there are signs of both motor and sensory involvement, although sometimes the symptomatology may be restricted to motor involvement (e.g. in lead poisoning). Polyneuropathies with predominantly sensory impairment occur as well (e.g. in diabetes, uraemia, myxoedema and leprosy). The condition can also manifest itself as a mononeuropathy (e.g. involvement of the n.femoralis in diabetes), or in the form of multiple mononeuropathies (in polyarteritis nodosa, leprosy or diabetes), or as a radiculopathy (e.g. Guillain–Barré syndrome and thoracic radiculopathy in diabetes).

The axon of the myelinated fibres is surrounded by a Schwann cell between the nodes of Ranvier. In some neuropathies the Schwann cell or the myelin sheath between two nodes of Ranvier are primarily affected (segmental demyelination). Other neuropathies predominantly show axonal involvement. This axonal degeneration usually commences in the most distal part of the nerve (dying-back phenomenon). Segmental demyelination occurs in neuropathies in diphtheria, chronic liver conditions, myxoedema, metachromatic leucodystrophy and globoid-cell leucodystrophy, among others. Axonal degeneration occurs, especially in toxic neuropathies, in polyneuropathies resulting from vitamin deficiency, and in neuropathies associated with porphyria. In many neuropathies there is both segmental demyelination and axonal degeneration (polyneuropathy in diabetes, uraemia, and in alcoholics).

In general the motor conduction velocity remains unaltered for a long time, and clinical recovery is very slow in the case of neuropathies with axonal degeneration. In neuropathies with segmental demyelination, on the other hand, motor conduction velocity is decreased from an early stage and recovery may be relatively quick. In some neuropathies granulomas may be observed between the nerve fibres (sarcoidosis) or there may be accumulations of abnormal substances (amyloid).

A vasculitis can cause ischaemia and give rise to neuropathies, in, for example, polyarteritis nodosa, lupus erythematosus, rheumatoid arthritis and other collagen diseases.

An enumeration of all disorders which may be associated with a neuropathy falls outside the scope of this book; however, various handbooks are available. In spite of the many chemicals known to trigger of toxic neuropathy (Table 7.1), it is not uncommon for an extensive examination to fail to establish a definite cause. In this chapter the diabetic neuropathies, polyneuropathy in alcoholics,

Table 7.1 Some causes of toxic neuropathies

Drugs,	
Anaesthetic	Trichlorethylene
Antibiotic	Streptomycin
	Sulphonamides
Anticonvulsive	Phenytoin
Antihypertensive	Hydralazine
Antimalarial	Chloroquine
Antiprotozoic	Emetine
	Metronidazole
Antimycotic	Amphotericin B
Alcoholism treatment	Disulfiram
Cytostatic	Ethoglucid
	Nitrogen mustard
	Vinblastine
	Vincristine
Intestinal	Clioquinol
Tuberculostatic	Isoniazid (INH)
Urinary-tract treatment	Nitrofurantoin

Heavy metals.
Antimony, arsenic, bismuth, gold, copper, mercury, lead, thallium.

Other substances.
Acrylamide, aniline, petrol, dinitrobenzene, dinitrophenol, carbon monoxide, triorthocresyl phosphate, carbon disulphide, ethylene oxide.

the Guillain–Barré syndrome and neuralgic amyotrophy will be discussed in more detail because they occur relatively frequently. Some hereditary neuropathies will be reviewed as well.

Diabetic neuropathies

The peripheral nerve can be affected in different ways in diabetes mellitus. Owing to this, numerous classifications have been made, most of which are impractical because the different syndromes often overlap. In general, a broad distinction can be made between the symmetric polyneuropathies on the one hand and the mononeuropathies (and multiple mononeuropathies) on the other (Table 7.2).

Table 7.2. Classification of the diabetic neuropathies.

Symmetric polyneuropathies.
(1) Distal, predominantly sensory polyneuropathy.
(2) Autonomic (visceral) neuropathy.

Mononeuropathy and multiple mononeuropathies.
(1) Isolated functional loss of peripheral nerves.
(2) Function loss of the cranial nerves.
(3) Diabetic amyotrophy.

The actual pathogenesis of diabetic neuropathy is not known. Both insulin deficiency and hyperglycaemia have been suggested as the cause of demyelination and axonal degeneration. In addition, it is likely that ischaemia of the nerve, caused by an obstruction of the small arteries, may play a role, especially in mononeuropathies. Although neuropathies can occur in well-stabilized and in poorly stabilized diabetics, they do seem to occur more often in the latter.

Diabetic polyneuropathy mainly occurs in patients between 50 and 60 years of age. There is a slow insidious onset with symptoms and signs based on sensory impairment in both the lower legs and feet. These sensory disturbances are sometimes the first clinical manifestation of diabetes. Patients complain of a dead feeling in their lower legs and feet, but paraesthesiae, hyperaesthesia and localized deep burning pains occur as well. Examination shows a marked loss of vibration sensation as well as absent ankle jerks. As a rule there is only a little, if any, bilateral muscular weakness in the lower legs and feet. Abnormalities are never found in the forearms and hands. If there is a serious loss of pain sensation, painless ulcers may develop on the soles of the feet. Arthropathies may also occur in the foot and ankle joints.

Autonomic (visceral) neuropathy

This is a form of diabetic neuropathy in which a variety of dysfunctions of the autonomic nervous system may occur, including little or no reaction of the pupils to light, nocturnal diarrhoea, anhidrosis, impotence, vasomotor disorders (orthostatic hypotension) and bladder disturbances (increased residual volume or sphincteric insufficiency).

Acute mononeuropathies and multiple mononeuropathies

These occur often, but as a rule their prognosis is more favourable than that of diabetic polyneuropathy. The vascular system is important in the development of these neuropathies. Although it is possible, in principle, for each peripheral nerve to be affected, the n.femoralis is most frequently involved one. The n.oculomotorius and the n.abducens are the most frequently affected cranial nerves. This often concerns patients older than 50 years of age. Symptoms are acute, usually occur on one side of the head, and are associated with pain. If the n.oculomotorius is affected, the innervation of the pupil appears to be almost always intact, which may be important for differential diagnosis.

Diabetic amyotrophy

This is more common in poorly stabilized diabetics of 50 years and older. Signs include an asymmetric weakness and wasting of the proximal muscles of the leg (m.quadriceps femoris, m.iliopsoas, hamstrings, adductors), and sometimes also of the mm.glutei. The signs are often preceded by severe pains in the upper leg. Knee jerks are absent as are signs of sensation impairment. There are electrophysiological and neuropathological indications of a proximal neuropathy and, frequently, an increased protein concentration in the cerebrospinal fluid—this prompts some authors to conclude that a radiculopathy is involved as well. In diabetics the disorder must be differentiated from a mononeuropathy of the n.femoralis in which the motor deficit is restricted to loss of the function of the m.quadriceps femoris and the m.iliopsoas.

Thoracic radiculopathy

This occurs in diabetics of 50 years of age and older. Severe pains in the front of the chest and abdomen develop gradually. The pain is indicated in an area of skin corresponding with one or more dermatomes, both uni- and bilateral. The corresponding areas of the back are sometimes painful as well. On examination of the painful areas there are sometimes hyperaesthesia and/or a reduction in pain sensation. The prognosis is good, but the pain may persist for months and sometimes years. Many patients have considerable weight loss, the cause of which remains unexplained.

Polyneuropathy in alcoholics

The exact pathogenesis of polyneuropathy in alcoholics is unknown. What is known is that an important role is played by an insufficient and one-sided diet (rich in carbohydrates). An alcoholic tends not only to skip meals but also to eat only bread, pasta and/or tinned soup. This gradually leads to a nutritional deficiency, particularly of thiamine and other vitamins. Many alcoholics have an asymptomatic polyneuropathy which only shows up on examination: slight signs of sensory dysfunction in the feet; less marked or absent ankle jerks and, sometimes, a sensitivity of the lower leg muscles under pressure. Furthermore, an electrophysiological examination will often show decreased motor and sensory nerve conduction velocities, especially distally.

When there are symptoms, these consist of muscle weakness and, less often, pain and paraesthesiae, distally, in the legs. The pain in the lower legs and feet can be continuous or episodic with severe shooting pains. In addition, patients also report a burning pain in the soles of the feet which varies in intensity and can get worse if touched.

Examination discloses symmetric pareses and atrophy, with the dorsal flexors of the feet and toes being particularly affected. Nevertheless, there are many patients who also show a mild weakness of the proximal muscles of the leg. If the condition has existed for a long time then weakness of the wrist and finger extensors is found as well. As a rule, the reflexes are lowered or absent: the latter applies particularly to the ankle jerks. Sensation is impaired and the area involved is sometimes stocking- or glove-shaped, its edges ill-defined so that there is a gradual transition to normal sensation. Histopathology shows both axons and myelin sheaths to be affected, with a preference for the distal parts of the nerves.

Therapy consists of stopping the use of alcohol and prescribing an adequate diet, rich in vitamins. If required, medication containing thiamine, pyridoxine, pantothenic acid and hydroxo-cobalamin may be administered. In addition, muscle-strengthening exercises and measures to prevent and control pes equinus should begin early. The prognosis will depend on whether or not the patient returns to alcohol abuse. If no alcohol is consumed and the therapeutic measures are carried out, the patient will enjoy a slow recovery.

Guillain–Barré syndrome

The Guillain–Barré or Guillain–Barré–Strohl syndrome manifests itself as an acute polyradiculoneuropathy. As a rule, the clinical signs appear 2 to 4 weeks after an aspecific respiratory-tract infection or gastrointestinal disorder ('influenza'). However, the syndrome has also been observed after diphtheria, herpes zoster, malaria, measles, parotitis, German measles and varicella. It has also been described after vaccinations and surgery. Its pathogenesis is unclear. In some cases antibodies against myelin are found in the serum. Neuropathologic examination shows segmental demyelina-tion and, in serious cases, axonal degeneration as well. There are also collections of lymphocytes in the perivascular spaces and in the interstitium, especially of the peripheral nerve roots. It is assumed that both the lymphocytes, which secrete a cytotoxic substance, and the macrophages play an important role in the destruction of myelin.

Paraesthesias of the feet, which spread proximally and may also occur in the hands, are the first symptom in approximately half the cases. This is followed by the development of a more or less symmetric muscle weakness which begins in the distal muscles and ascends to the proximal muscles, first in the legs (especially the hamstrings) and later in the arms as well. The severity of the muscle involvement may vary from very slight muscle weakness in the lower legs to a total paralysis of all limbs. If the diaphragm and the intercostal muscles become involved, serious respiratory insufficiency will develop. Facial palsy, sometimes bilateral, occurs in 50 per cent of patients. Other cranial nerves may be involved as well: the n.oculomotorius, n.trochlearis, n.abducens, n.glossopharyngeus, and the n.hypoglossus. The condition begins with cranial nerve impairment in about 5 per cent of patients. The Miller–Fisher syndrome, which is accompanied by ophthalmoplegia, ataxia, and areflexia, is a separate variant.

Signs of involvement of the autonomic nervous system occur regularly, although their intensity often varies: arrhythmias, attacks of tachycardia, hypertension, orthostatic hypotension, hyperhidrosis, impairment of pupil reaction (usually a sluggish reaction to stimulation by light), urine retention or intestinal atony. The reflexes are weak or absent, except for the abdominal reflexes which usually remain intact.

Signs of sensory impairment do not predominate although impaired perception of vibration and of movements of the joints may occur. In classic cases a marked increase in the protein content of the cerebrospinal fluid (up to 2 g/100 ml), the cell count remaining normal, occurs about 1 week after the first signs have appeared. After several weeks about 80 per cent of the patients have reduced motor nerve conduction velocities. However, a correlation between the severity of this loss of conduction and the degree of the pareses does not exist. A stationary phase in the clinical picture is reached within 2 to 4 weeks; after this a gradual, though often only partial, recovery takes place in the following months. A recurrent and a chronic form of the syndrome also exists.

In serious cases there is always the threat of respiratory dysfunction and acute respiratory failure. For that reason regular monitoring of the vital capacity is necessary, and artificial ventilation should be available. Therapy is symptomatic and includes the prevention and control of contractures and decubitus and the treatment of autonomic dysfunction such as hypertension and arrhythmia. Corticosteroids have little effect, if any, on the course of the syndrome. Favourable results, however, are sometimes obtained with the administration of plasma, especially in chronic cases.

Neuralgic amyotrophy

Neuralgic amyotrophy is also known as brachial plexus neuropathy or shoulder-girdle neuritis. The condition became known in the Second World War as it occurred frequently among the Allied troops. Men are more often affected than women (3:1). In about half the patients, the condition follows an infectious disease, but the symptoms may also occur after an operation or trauma. The interval between exposure to the triggering factor and the onset of symptoms and signs is usually 4 to 5 days and rarely longer than 2 weeks.

The pathogenesis of the syndrome is unclear. Although vascular disorders, allergies and viruses are suspected, no cause can be found in half the patients. The condition begins with pain on one side of the shoulder girdle. Some patients experience no pain; in others, the pain may occur acutely at night, or in the morning on waking, and can persist for days or weeks. A paresis or even paralysis of the m.serratus anterior, the m.supraspinatus, the m.infraspinatus, the m.trapezius and the m.deltoideus develop several hours or days after the pain. These muscles waste relatively rapidly. Other muscle groups are hardly ever affected. Involvement of the m.serratus anterior (n.thoracalis longus) appears to be preferred and the shoulder muscles on the other side of the body may become involved in a minority of cases. If the process is unilateral, electromyographical abnormalities in the clinically unaffected shoulder musculature (e.g. fibrillation potentials and positive sharp waves) may be found.

Sensation disturbances are not prominent. Sometimes there is hypaesthesia in the region of the skin innervated by the n.axillaris. The cerebrospinal fluid is normal as a rule.

The patient's prognosis is generally favourable, regardless of location and degree of the muscle weakness. The muscle weakness begins to recover after 9 to 12 months. Approximately 80 per cent of the patients will recover within 2 years and 90 per cent will have fully recovered in 3. Therapy is symptomatic: treatment of pain in the acute phase and the use of passive movements to prevent contractures of the shoulder joint. When making a differential diagnosis, the hereditary brachial plexus neuropathy should be considered; this is an autosomal dominant disease with varying expressivity. In some families the sufferers show hypotelorism. In addition, it is necessary to exclude other processes in the brachial plexus. The brachial plexus neuritis which occurs in serum sickness and after vaccination is clinically very similar to neuralgic amyotrophy. The patient's history of this basically rare complication will, of course, lead to the correct diagnosis.

Hereditary motor and sensory neuropathies

The hereditary motor and sensory neuropathies (HMSN) form a group of diseases which used collectively to be called Charcot–Marie–Tooth disease. Nowadays, improvements in electrophysiological technique and in the pathology of nerve biopsies have made it easier to distinguish between these clinically very similar conditions. However, there is no generally accepted classification of these neuropathies (Table 7.3). There are both dominant and recessive forms and either may be accompanied by segmental demyelination (type I) or axonal degeneration (type II). The gene of type-I HMSN is located at the long arm of chromosome 1. In segmental demyelination (and remyelination) the axon remains unaffected and 'onion-bulb' formation occurs as a result of the hyperplasia of Schwann cells. In axonal degeneration the axon is primarily affected and any lesion of the myelin sheath is secondary. Regeneration (sprouting) may occur but there is no 'onion-bulb' formation. The HMSN can also be classified on the basis of motor nerve conduction velocities. Here the conduction of the n.medianus is especially important: if it is below 38 m/second it suggests type I and, if above, type II. This figure, however, depends not only upon the method used for determining the conduction velocity but also on the temperature at the nerve. It is also important to remember that the clinical picture of distal spinal muscular atrophy is very similar to that of the HMSN types, and for that reason it should always be kept in mind as a differential diagnostic alternative.

The signs usually commence in the lower legs. Patients may complain of muscle cramp in their calves, and fasciculations are sometimes present.

Both symptoms tend to disappear as the disease progresses. Foot deformities such as talipes equinovarus, clawed toes (see Fig. 7.1) and, usually, pes cavus as well, develop because the small

Table 7.3. The main differences between hereditary motor and sensory neuropathies.

HMSN type I

Hypertrophic neuropathy of the Charcot–Marie–Tooth type.
Usually autosomal dominant, sometimes autosomal recessive or sporadic.
Onset often in childhood.
Forearms and hands are paretic in about 70 per cent of patients.
Sensory impairment in about 70 per cent of patients.
Motor and sensory conduction velocities are markedly decreased.
Segmental demyelination of the nerve with 'onion-bulb' formation.

HMSN type II

Neuronal form of the Charcot–Marie–Tooth type.
Autosomal dominant or recessive; rarely X-linked recessive.
Onset often around the age of 20 years, but also much later.
Forearms and hands are paretic in about 50 per cent of patients.
Sensory impairment in about 40 per cent of the patients.
Motor and sensory conduction velocities are slightly decreased.
Axonal degeneration.

HMSN type III

Hypertrophic neuropathy of the Déjérine–Sottas type.
Rare variant of type I.
Always autosomal recessive or sporadic.
Congenitally present or onset in the first years of life.
Severe course.
Marked demyelination (hypomyelination) and many 'onion bulbs'.

The main disease to be differentiated from HMSN types I and II is *Distal spinal muscular atrophy*.

Autosomal dominant, recessive or sporadic.
Onset in childhood, but also in later life.
Forearms and hands are paretic in approximately 25 per cent of patients.
No impairment of sensation.
Motor and sensory conduction velocities are normal.
No hypertrophy, demyelination or axonal degeneration of the nerve.

---

muscles of the foot (especially the m.extensor digitorum brevis) become involved at an early stage. These patients are often first seen and treated by an orthopaedic surgeon with foot-arch supports and/or special footwear. Gradually, however, the picture

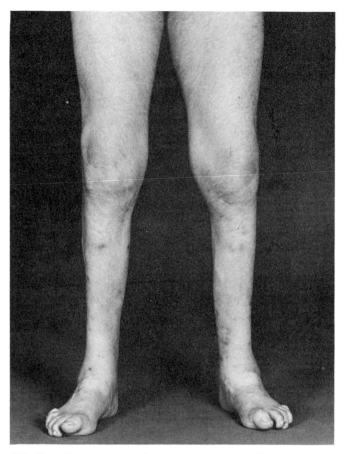

Fig. 7.1. Hereditary motor and sensory neuropathy (type I). There is a marked discrepancy between the circumference of the lower and upper legs as a result of severe wasting of the foot and toe extensors. The toes are clawed.

becomes clearer with weakness and wasting developing in the m.tibialis anterior, the toe extensors and the mm.peroneus longus and brevis (Fig. 7.1). For that reason the disease used to be called 'peroneal muscular atrophy'. Later the muscles of the calves also weaken and waste (Fig. 7.2). Although some wasting of the distal third part of the upper leg muscles may also occur in some patients, what is noticeable in the first instance is the sometimes very strong dissimilarity between the circumference of the lower and upper leg. In this context they are sometimes called 'stork legs', an aspect which in any case can only be observed clearly in a minority of patients (especially in type II).

If the symptomatology extends at a later stage to the upper limbs, then difficulties with fine finger movement (doing up buttons etc.) often form the first symptom. The m.interosseus I and II are affected first, followed by the muscles of the thenar and hypothenar (Fig. 7.3 and 7.4), and finally the finger flexors.

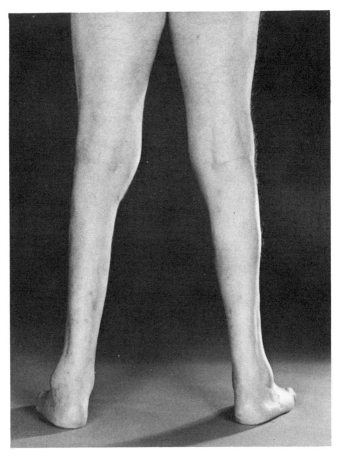

Fig. 7.2. Hereditary motor and sensory neuropathy. The calf muscles also atrophy at a later stage of the disease.

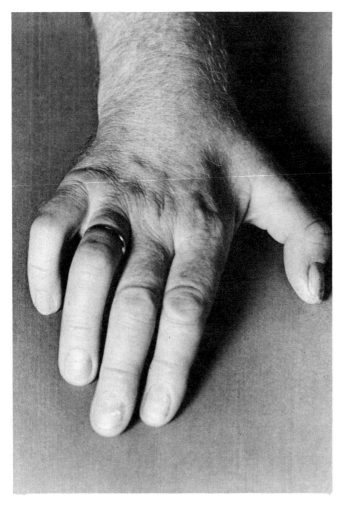

Fig. 7.3. Hereditary motor and sensory neuropathy (type I). There is wasting of the m.interosseus primus as well as flexion contracture of the fingers.

Generally the extensors are only slightly affected, if at all. Since the onset of the process is gradual and further progression particularly slow (years!), the patient has ample opportunity to adapt to his handicap. It is often remarkable how much the patient can still do with his hands despite severe weakness and wasting.

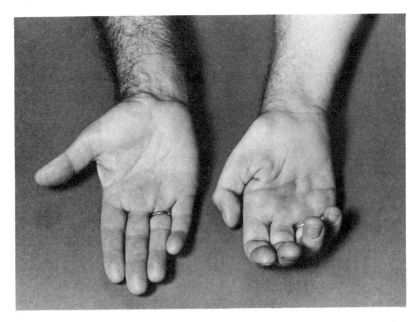

Fig. 7.4. Hereditary motor and sensory neuropathy (type I). Atrophy of the thenar and hypothenar. Flexion contracture of the fingers. Healthy hand on the left, for comparison.

This is very different for a patient with, for example, a traumatic lesion of the n.ulnaris or with a rapidly progressive polyneuropathy of the hands and who is then seriously handicapped by the accompanying motor disorder. Flexion contractures of the fingers occur in only a minority of cases, usually in patients with HMSN type I (see Figs. 7.3 and 7.4). The symptomatology of the disease is bilateral although often asymmetric: initially the patient may only complain of a footdrop on one side, but subsequent examination will show that the other side is involved as well, albeit to a lesser degree. This difference in severity of the weakness may persist for many years.

The ankle jerks generally disappear and the knee jerks are reduced or absent in about 50 per cent of patients. If the forearms are strongly affected as well, then the radial and ulnar reflexes may become negative. The plantar reflexes are normal, although often impossible to assess because of the severe muscle weakness and foot deformation. The vibration sensation is often impaired, touch and pain sensations less so, and the joint position sensation even less. In approximately 25 per cent of the patients with type I, hypertrophy of the nerve can lead to clinically verifiable enlarged peripheral nerves, especially the peroneal nerves, but others too, such as the n.auricularis magnus. Every experienced neurologist, however, knows how difficult it is to conclude on the basis of palpation whether or not a peroneal nerve is enlarged.

Sometimes other signs can be observed, for example, involvement of the upper motor neuron (HMSN type V), atrophy of the optic nerves (HMSN type VI), pigment degeneration of the retina (HMSN type VII), and tremor and ataxia (Roussy–Lévy syndrome), kyphoscoliosis, anisocoria, deafness, and cardiac conduction disturbances. All these combinations of peroneal muscular atrophy are also known as the 'complicated Charcot–Marie–Tooth syndrome'. In this respect one could also speak of 'HMSN-plus'. There are still other diseases (Refsum's disease, spinocerebellar degenerations, myotonic dystrophy, etc.) which may be accompanied by weakness and wasting of the muscles innervated by the peroneal nerves. It is not possible to differentiate between HMSN types I and II on the basis of clinical data. This always requires additional examinations in which the determination of motor and sensory conduction velocities is especially important. A biopsy from the sural nerve also contributes to the diagnosis. Besides, it must be realized that a hypertrophic neuropathy with 'onion-bulb' formation is not specific to HMSN types I or III but can also occur in other polyneuropathies, for example those due to diabetes. Serum creatine kinase is usually normal while a muscle biopsy reveals neurogenic abnormalities but is unable to contribute to a further differentiation of the disease.

No therapy is available for the hereditary motor and sensory neuropathies. Genetic counselling, however, plays an important role in preventing the disease. It must be borne in mind that autosomal dominant forms may show a marked variety of gene expression so that the heterozygotes may only show minimal signs. Indeed, it is possible that the only sign is decreased motor conduction velocity of the peripheral nerves. For this reason it is always necessary to subject both parents to a careful neurological and electrophysiological examination before giving genetic advice. A symptomatic treatment with physiotherapy can noticeably prolong the patient's mobility in this very slowly progressive disease. Suitable footwear and, at a more advanced stage, an ankle–foot arthrodesis can also be of great help to the patient. The extent to which these patients require foot surgery, especially lengthening of the Achilles tendons, is questioned. Generally, the results of such operations have been disappointing. Although each case has of course to be judged on its own merits it seems good practice to postpone surgery for as long as possible.

Hereditary neuropathy with liability to pressure palsies

This hereditary neuropathy manifests itself as an increased sensitivity of the peripheral nerves to external compression. The resulting pareses usually recover in the next few days or weeks. The disease is autosomal dominant and probably occurs more often than is generally assumed. Approximately half the patients suffer from pes cavus.

In principle, it is possible for every peripheral nerve, and sometimes a cranial nerve as well, to be temporarily affected by mechanical influences. There appears to be a preference however, for the peroneal nerve at the level of the fibular head, for the radial, ulnaris, and median nerves, and the brachial plexus. If the nerve is compressed repeatedly, residual effects may persist. The peroneal nerve becomes involved in patients who have persistently squatted or knelt at work; the disease has been described in workers lifting bulbs and potatoes. Sitting with the knees crossed for prolonged periods may also cause peroneal palsy. The first symptoms sometimes consist of paraesthesiae in the lower leg and foot, but the patient does not complain of pain. Signs of motor and sensory involvement, which the patient will first experience as a footdrop, then develop. Peripheral nerve impairment may also occur as a consequence of, for instance, pressure during narcosis, plaster on the lower leg, knee bandages, labour, etc.

Motor and sensory nerve conduction velocities are frequently decreased, not only in the clinically affected nerve but also in clinically healthy peripheral nerves. By means of these electrophysiological methods one can often recognize heterozygotes who have never had a pressure palsy before. Apart from the family history, the demonstration of sausage-like enlargements (tomacula) of the myelinated fibres in a biopsy of the sural nerve is very important in establishing the correct diagnosis.

Postscript

There are few drugs which can cure a neuropathy, but many which can cause one.

Although the vitamin B complex plays an important role in the neuronal metabolism of a normally functioning nerve, there are no grounds for assuming that vitamin B has a stimulating effect on the regeneration of a diseased nerve.

Neuropathies based on a vitamin B deficiency are relatively rare. Doctors who do not prescribe vitamin B for every neuropathy are still rarer.

A neuropathy can also occur in stabilized diabetics.

Not every neuropathy which occurs in a diabetic patient is caused by diabetes.

The Guillain–Barré syndrome is a very benign condition: the patient may be cured completely.

The Guillain–Barré syndrome is a very serious condition: the patient requires artificial ventilation.

In many neuropathies a nerve biopsy contributes little to the diagnosis. Muscle biopsies usually contribute even less in such cases.

The condition which was earlier called Charcot–Marie–Tooth disease or peroneal muscular atrophy is now called HMSN. Despite the many names and numerous classifications, the clinical picture of this disease has not changed.

The hereditary motor and sensory neuropathies are not always hereditary.

Not all hereditary motor and sensory neuropathies show sensory disturbances.

Decreased motor conduction velocities of the peripheral nerves may be the only abnormality in HMSN, which is important in identifying heterozygotes (and also therefore, in genetic counselling).

If a patient with HMSN wants to stay on his feet as long as possible, foot surgery must be postponed as long as possible.

8
Myasthenia gravis

Myasthenia gravis belongs to the group of diseases which are related by a defect in neuromuscular transmission. It is a non-hereditary disease characterized by variability in muscular weakness. This muscle weakness worsens or is provoked by exercise of the muscle or muscle groups involved, while rest leads to an improvement. The location and clinical course of this muscle weakness vary a great deal.

Myasthenia gravis can occur at any age. Most authors report that the condition is two to three times more prevalent in women than in men. Weakness of the extraocular muscles is the first manifestation of this disease in about 60 per cent of the patients. The disease can also commence with bulbar phenomena (about 20 per cent of cases), or with muscle weakness in the extremities. It is generally assumed that the first signs can be precipitated by excessive muscular exercise, infectious diseases, surgery, and the puerperium, as well as by strong emotions and stress. Double vision is often the first complaint when the extraocular muscles are involved. It usually first occurs in the evening after a tiring day at work and, initially, disappears again the next morning. Gradually, however, the patient begins to notice that double vision occurs more often, increases during the day, and is still there — even after a night's sleep — the next morning. Ptosis of one or both eyelids may occur as well. A bilateral ptosis is almost always asymmetric and fluctuating. In a number of patients (10–15 per cent) the myasthenic symptoms remain limited to the extraocular muscles.

Dysarthria, dysphagia, and difficulties with mastication may occur if the bulbar, innervated muscles are affected. If the patient talks for a long time, the voice may begin to sound nasal and become dysarthric. Later still, the voice becomes steadily softer, and eventually the patient can no longer be understood. During meals there is difficulty with mastication and sometimes the patient has to put his hand under his chin to compensate for the weakened chewing movements. Dysphagia may lead to considerable weight loss. If the facial muscles are affected, the face often takes on a totally different expression. People think that the patient always looks sad, sour, or angry, and they are strengthened in their opinion by the fact that when laughing the patient will pull up his upper lip as if he is about to cry. The neck muscles may also weaken, making it difficult to balance the head. The patient tries to compensate for this by supporting his head with a hand. The disease affects the arms more often than the legs and the proximal muscles more often than the distal musculature. Reflexes are always normal.

Muscular atrophy, as a result of denervation, only occurs in about 10 per cent of patients; it is located in the shoulder girdle, the upper arms, the face, and tongue. The tongue sometimes has three longitudinal furrows, a sign which is considered to be very characteristic of myasthenia gravis, although it rarely occurs.

The muscle weakness can often only be identified or provoked by inducing extra effort for the muscles involved. Thus, the patient could be asked to look sideways or upwards for at least half a minute to precipitate ptosis and diplopia. According to some authors, an even better way of stimulating ptosis than asking the patient to look up, is to ask him to abduct the eyes. Diplopia can also be caused by provoking an optokinetic nystagmus for 1 minute. Ptosis can sometimes be induced by getting the patient to look into a bright light. Dysarthria can be provoked by getting the patient to count or read aloud from a book. Dysfunction of the masseter muscles can be provoked by the mouth being opened and firmly (and audibly) closed a number of times in rapid succession. Healthy people easily manage to do this 100 times within half a minute. Weakness of the neck flexors can be provoked by asking the supine patient to lift his head and watch his navel for 1 minute. Weakness of the shoulder girdle and arm musculature can be provoked by asking the patient to stretch his arms, hands and fingers in front of him for 3 minutes. One way of provoking leg-muscle weakness is to ask the patient to make many successive deep knee bends (at least 20 times is normally possible), to walk on his heels or toes (normally at least 30 steps should be possible) or to raise his leg to a 45 degree angle when supine (this can normally be kept up for at least one minute).

The pathogenesis of myasthenia gravis is not fully known. Under normal circumstances, a nerve impulse will cause acetylcholine to be released into the synaptic cleft. The acetylcholine subsequently diffuses through this cleft and connects with the acetylcholine receptors, which are situated at the top of the post-synaptic folds of the motor end-plates. The acetylcholine action is interrupted by the enzyme acetylcholinesterase, which hydrolyses the acetylcholine to acetic acid and choline. In myasthenia gravis this neuromuscular transmission is impaired owing to a substantial loss in the number of acetylcholine receptors (only 20–30 per cent of the normal amount). Furthermore, the synaptic cleft is widened and the number of post-synaptic folds reduced as well. Owing to the reduction in the number of acetylcholine receptors it is no longer possible for normal, or even increased, concentrations of acetylcholine to have an optimal effect. The first impulses usually produce enough acetylcholine to cause a muscle contraction, but the subsequent impulses release increasingly smaller quantities. The receptors are now no longer stimulated and polarization of the muscle fibre membrane does not take place. As a result a growing number of muscle fibres become blocked and are no longer able to participate in muscle contraction. It is clear, therefore, that anticholinesterases will have a favourable effect on myasthenia gravis because they inhibit the breakdown of acetylcholine by acetylcholinesterase, enabling more acetylcholine to be available following a nerve impulse. However, if too many anticholinesterases are given, too much acetylcholine may well inactivate the receptors and cause further muscle weakness (cholinergic crisis). Serum antibodies against acetylcholine receptors are found in approximately 90 per cent of the patients with myasthenia gravis. These antibodies are very specific for myasthenia. They may be absent, however; this occurs in about half of the patients with ocular myasthenia gravis.

The thymus plays an important although far from understood role in the pathogenesis of myasthenia gravis. Both hyperplasia and germinal centres occur in about 70 per cent of patients. It is remarkable that a thymoma occurs in about 10 per cent of the patients (and in as many as 30 per cent of those over 40 years of age). Most myasthenia patients with a thymoma have antibodies against cross-striated muscle tissue. Hyperplasia of the thymus and the absence of a normal thymus involution occur in about three-quarters of those without thymoma. This particularly concerns young patients.

The diagnosis of myasthenia gravis is based on the patient's history (fluctuations in muscle weakness) and the testing of muscle power after exercise, which either provokes or aggravates the muscular weakness.

There are several other tests which can suggest or confirm the diagnosis. As mentioned earlier, antibodies against acetylcholine receptor proteins are very characteristic, and for that reason their identification is most important for the diagnosis. A diagnosis can also be made more likely by administering anticholinesterases (atropine–neostigmine test, Table 8.1). The so-called curare test is only justified in reaching a diagnosis when administered by a specialist, and then only under certain circumstances. Electrophysiology can also be used to support the diagnosis. If supramaximal stimuli with a frequency of 1–3 per second are given to the motor nerve, the effect of the muscle action-potential (AP) produced can be recorded by a surface electrode. The first AP is usually normal, but subsequent APs will become progressively reduced, reaching a minimum at the fifth. A reduction of at least 10 per cent is typical of myasthenia gravis. Other electrophysiological phenomena (post-tetanic potentiation, post-tetanic exhaustion) and methods (single-fibre electromyography) can also be

Table 8.1. The atropine–neostigmine test.

---

(1) First administer 0.5 mg atropine i.m. Wait five minutes. If the muscular weakness improves, then this is a placebo effect.

(2) Administer 1.5–2.0 mg neostigmine (methylsulphate) i.m. If the test is positive the muscular weakness improves or disappears after 10–15 minutes. This effect will last from an hour to an hour and a half.

(3) If the test is negative: repeat it at the end of the day after strenuous muscular exercise.

---

employed when trying to establish the existence of impaired neuromuscular transmission.

A muscle biopsy contributes little to the diagnosis: type-II-fibre atrophy, signs of denervation, and round cell infiltrates (lymphorrhages) may occur, but as a rule the biopsy is normal. One can of course find abnormalities if the biopsy is taken from the end-plate zone and examined by intravital methylene blue staining (elongated end-plates) or by electron microscopy (widened primary synaptic clefts, few and often shallow secondary synaptic clefts).

The treatment of myasthenia gravis consists of the administration of anticholinesterases. Pyridostigmine bromide in a dose of 20–120 mg orally 5 to 6 times a day should be considered first. Adverse side-effects such as diarrhoea, stomach complaints, and hypersalivation usually disappear after a few weeks or can be treated with atropine sulphate orally (⅛ to ¼ mg 5 to 6 times a day). If necessary, other drugs (neostigmine bromide, ephedrine hydrochloride) can be given as well. Women whose symptoms and signs get worse during the premenstrual period may benefit from taking oral contraceptives. The beneficial effects of anticholinesterases usually decrease after a few months (probably because the disease is progressive) so the dose must be increased. Nevertheless, it can be said that most patients improve considerably as a result of careful treatment with anticholinesterases even though the muscles never recover entirely.

Treatment with prednisone must be considered, especially for patients who are older than 50 years and have severe generalized myasthenia. Older patients with ocular myasthenia can react very well to prednisone if insufficient results are obtained with the usual methods (covering the eye, mechanical correction of the ptosis, and so on). Initially, it is recommended that 25 mg prednisone be given on alternate days and that the dose be increased, by 5 mg up to 100 mg, on alternate days. After approximately two months the dose can be reduced again (by 2.5 mg a week) until an optimal dose is achieved (usually 30–50 mg every other day). If a higher dose than 50 mg prednisone every other day seems necessary, then azathioprine can be added (50 mg per day, to be increased gradually to 150 mg per day), as a result of which the prednisone dose can be reduced. Treatment with azathioprine alone can also achieve favourable results. If no spontaneous remission has occurred within a year, then a thymectomy is indicated in all patients with generalized myasthenia between 10 and 40 years of age, irrespective of whether they responded to treatment with anticholinesterases or not. A thymectomy leads to a remission within three years in 30 per cent of the patients between 10 and 40 years of age, whereas there is only a 10 per cent likelihood of this happening spontaneously. Thymectomy is also indicated for patients between 40 and 50 years of age who have a generalized myasthenia, have not responded to anticholinesterases, and who have had the disease for less than three years. In fact, the indications for thymectomy vary enormously between countries and clinics. Any existing thymoma must be removed because of the possibility of invasive growth. Plasma exchange must be considered, especially in patients with acute respiratory distress, or as a preparation for thymectomy in seriously weakened patients.

A sudden deterioration of the muscle weakness and respiratory difficulties (myasthenic crisis) occurs in approximately 20 per cent of patients with generalized myasthenia. Such a crisis is said to occur in as many as 50 per cent of the patients with thymoma. The crisis is often heralded by short attacks of dyspnoea, an increased difficulty in swallowing, tachycardia, hypertension, restlessness, and insomnia. During the crisis the patient is anxious and often has dilated pupils, heavy perspiration, over-secretion of saliva, tachycardia, and the urge to urinate and defaecate. A myasthenic crisis is difficult to distinguish from a — actually rare — cholinergic crisis. The latter develops in myasthenic patients who have received a (relative) overdose of anticholinesterases. Such patients always show narrowed pupils. One must be alert to the fact that the increase in muscle weakness of a myasthenic patient leads to incremental dosing and, finally, to overdosing with anti-cholinesterases. This leads to a combination of myasthenic crisis and cholinergic crisis. The treatment of a cholinergic crisis (high-dose atropine, 1–8 mg i.v.) or myasthenic crisis can only start if the patient has been admitted to an intensive-care unit with artificial ventilation facilities. Myasthenic crisis is best treated by administering 100 mg prednisone per day for a period of 3 weeks. These patients tend to get myasthenic crises more than once.

The course of the disease is often erratic and hard to predict. Spontaneous fluctuations occur, but the clinical picture can also be influenced by infectious diseases, endocrine factors (menstruation, pregnancy, menopause) or emotion and stress. Various drugs can have an adverse effect on muscle weakness; these include diazepam, phenytoin, neomycin, streptomycin, acetazolamide, quinidine, procainamide, penicillamine, propranolol, and other beta-blockers. In general, the disease reaches its peak after 3 to 5 years, at which time the signs show little change in intensity and hardly any new signs appear. Ocular myasthenia has a relatively benign course, the signs remaining limited to the extraocular muscles.

A separate place must be reserved for neonatal myasthenia, which occurs in about 12 per cent of the children delivered of myasthenic mothers. The first signs appear between several hours and 3 days after birth. There is general muscle weakness and difficulty with sucking and swallowing, while crying is weak. Ptosis, strabismus and facial weakness may sometimes occur as well. It is important to recognize respiratory disorders, as they may lead to the child's death. The signs disappear again after several weeks or sometimes even two months. Treatment consists of careful nursing, the administration of anticholinesterases, and artificial ventilation if required.

Postscript

A history of fluctuating muscular weakness and its demonstration during examination (by provoking it by muscular exercise) form the key to the diagnosis of myasthenia gravis. As usual, forgetting the key leads to a lot of discomfort.

Chronic tiredness is hardly ever due to myasthenia gravis.

Not every patient with fluctuating eye muscle weakness has myasthenia gravis.

Not every patient with myasthenia gravis has eye muscle weakness.

Most good neurologists have sometimes thought of hysteria in a patient with myasthenia.

Most good neurologists have sometimes thought of myasthenia in a patient with hysteria.

9

The Lambert–Eaton syndrome

In the Lambert–Eaton syndrome less acetylcholine than normal is released at the peripheral nerve ends. The patients complain of fatigued muscles (especially those of the legs) and show a proximal weakness which especially affects the pelvic girdle and upper leg musculature. After rest (e.g. in the morning on getting up) muscle power is very limited, but it increases again after some exercise; then, as the day progresses, it diminishes once more. The extraocular and bulbar muscles are seldom affected although some ptosis may occur. In addition, the patients complain of muscle pain and paraesthesiae in the hands and feet. As the myotatic reflexes are often decreased or absent it is assumed that a light neuropathy is also involved. Parasympathetic dysfunctions, such as dry mouth, obstipation, bladder disturbances, and impotence, are frequent. The syndrome occurs predominantly in men over 40 years of age and about 70 per cent of them will have a malignant condition, usually a bronchial tumour (oat-cell carcinoma) as well.

Electromyography reveals that the evoked action potential has a very low amplitude after supramaximal stimulation of the nerve. This amplitude will diminish further with low-frequency stimulation (1–3 Hz). The amplitude increases sharply, 4 to 20 times higher than its baseline value, after high-frequency stimulation (10–50 Hz). The initially very low amplitude of the action potential can also increase as a result of voluntary muscle contractions.

Guanidine (500 mg, 3–4 times per day) is the preferred drug. Prednisone, azathioprine, and plasma exchange are alternatives. The response of the weak muscles to anticholinesterases is only modest. The removal of any existing tumour does not usually have a favourable effect on muscle weakness.

10

Duchenne muscular dystrophy

Duchenne muscular dystrophy is probably the best known myopathy, so much so, in fact, that often the more general term 'muscular dystrophy' is used when referring to Duchenne muscular dystrophy. It is certainly not one of the most frequent neuromuscular diseases, but its course is among the most dramatic. The disease is X-linked recessive. The gene for Duchenne muscular dystrophy is located at the short arm of the X chromosome. Most authors think that in about 30 per cent of cases the disease is caused by spontaneous mutation, either in the mother's ovum or in the fertilized egg. Others, however, report a low rate of mutation, and they suggest that every mother of a son with Duchenne muscular dystrophy should be considered a carrier until the opposite is proven.

Although the cause of the disease is unknown, there are three theories about its pathogenesis, namely, a myogenic or membrane theory, a vascular theory and a neurogenic theory.

Electron microscopy has shown that one of the first abnormalities in the muscle fibre is formed by a wedge-shaped lesion. This causes local disruption of the inner plasma membrane. However, freeze-fracture studies of the muscle plasma membrane revealed abnormalities on both sides of the membrane. Numerous biochemical, enzyme, and morphological abnormalities in the erythrocyte membrane have also been described. For that reason it was initially thought that Duchenne muscular dystrophy was an expression of a more generalized membrane defect. As the findings could not always be reproduced or confirmed, many authors still wonder whether such a general membrane defect might not exist. The vascular theory is based mainly on the similarity between the histopathological findings of the muscle in Duchenne muscular dystrophy and those observed in rabbits and rats with induced experimental muscle ischaemia. Other researchers were, however, unable to show any defects in the microcirculation of the muscle in Duchenne muscular dystrophy, while electron microscopy could not find any relevant changes of the small arterial vessels and capillaries either. In the early sixties it was suggested, on the basis of electrophysiological findings, that in Duchenne muscular dystrophy there were 'sick' motor neurons. Numerous, particularly morphologic, investigations have made this neurogenic theory extremely unlikely.

Some infant patients are silent and move very little while still in the cradle. In most cases though, the first clinical signs appear when the child shows delayed motor development. He is late sitting, standing and walking and when he does begin to walk, he often falls. Young children with Duchenne muscular dystrophy who are just beginning to walk will often have facial injuries and many bruises. The parents notice how difficult it is for the child to get up again once it has fallen. Initially, this is explained away by the parents as 'laziness' or 'clumsiness'. Some patients do not learn to walk unsupported before they are 2 years old; these children rarely learn to run fast. Owing to the late walking development and the different walking pattern the parents come to realize that something is wrong with their son. Even then it may still take many years before the correct diagnosis is established. The main reason for this is that the doctors consulted do not usually recognize the often slight clinical signs, and then frequently deny them and reassure the parents. The patient is often referred to an orthopaedic surgeon because many physicians seem to think of foot deformations when observing walking disorders. As many of the patients will have flat feet as well, arch supports are often prescribed. The time between the first consultation and establishing the correct diagnosis can vary from 0–8 years, with an average of 3 years. By that time the patient's mean age is 6.

As so often in medicine, the diagnosis is easy once it is thought of. After listening carefully to the mother and not dismissing her concern about her child as 'excessive worry', inspection of the child may provide a great deal of information. In such cases further neurological examination does not really contribute very much to the diagnosis, especially since the possibility of testing isolated muscles in such young children is limited. First, it is obvious that the child stands with its abdomen forward and has hyperlordosis. On inspection, relatively well developed or even hypertrophic calf muscles are observed (Fig. 10.1). From a genuine compensatory hypertrophy, this will develop into a pseudohypertrophy, large parts of the degenerated muscle tissue

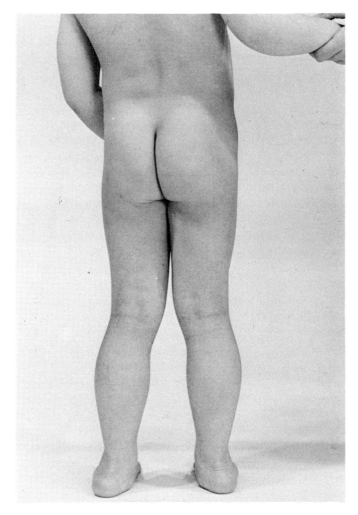

Fig. 10.1. Duchenne muscular dystrophy. The calf muscles are hypertrophied. The patient stands on the inside of his feet (pedes valgi).

being replaced by fatty and connective tissues. At an early stage in the disease the calf muscles feel firm on palpation. Often the patient has flat feet as well, with the tendency to rest on the inner side of the foot when standing or walking. Genua recurvata can also be observed. Scapulae alatae may be present, but it is often very difficult to conclude whether some degree of winging of the shoulders at this age is truly pathological. Many healthy young boys can show this phenomenon.

There is an unmistakable waddling gait when walking as well as a frequent tendency to abduct the arms to make balancing easier. In more advanced stages a tendency to stand and walk on tiptoe can be noted, and the child is unable to walk on his heels. If he is asked to run fast, he cannot, nor can he jump in the air from a standing position. Gowers' sign (see p. 16) can be observed when the child is asked to lie on his back on the floor and then get up. In fact, this is not specific for Duchenne muscular dystrophy; it occurs in all neuromuscular diseases involving a weakness of the hip extensors. It is, on the other hand, a very early sign in Duchenne muscular dystrophy. The child is also unable to rise from a low chair without pushing himself up with his hands. If the patient is asked to climb stairs, it will be noted that he prefers or finds it easier using both hands and feet. If he attempts to do this when upright, he will invariably use the same leg to negotiate each step, pulling the other leg up alongside before taking the next step. He will also rely heavily on his arms to pull himself up using the bannisters.

Neurological examination shows more weakness in the pelvic girdle and leg musculature than in the muscles of the shoulder girdle and arms. The patellar reflexes are often poor or absent. At a later stage the arm reflexes disappear as well; the ankle reflexes disappear last. Between the ages of 3 and 6 normal growth and development of the muscular system and an increase in motor skills will often compensate for the progressive degeneration, so that it seems as if the process has halted or an improvement in muscular function has taken place. This sometimes gives the parents false hope and they think that the doctor has made an incorrect diagnosis. The child might also have had 'alternative' medical treatment during this period. Thus, any improvement noted will serve as irrefutable proof that alternative therapy works. Many patients will continue to walk and climb stairs reasonably well until they are 8 years old. Then these functions deteriorate rapidly, because of an increase in the contractures of the iliotibial bands and the Achilles tendons. The process continues gradually and, in time, many other muscles weaken. There may be slight involvement of the facial musculature, but the extraocular and bulbar muscles always remain unaffected. By about the age of 11 most patients require a wheelchair. The flexion contractures of the elbows, hips and knees then deteriorates and the feet often become fixed in an equinovarus position. Sometimes a serious kyphoscoliosis develops. Contractures in the shoulder joints take a remarkably long time to develop. During these years many of these patients become fairly obese, although this is definitely not the rule. Pulmonary and sometimes cardiac complications finally prove fatal, although survival has been increased owing to the use of antibiotics and better treatment available for respiratory difficulties; in general, however, it is rare for these patients to reach the age of 30.

Cardiomyopathy occurs in over 80 per cent of the patients. Its clinical manifestations include heart enlargement, signs of decompensation, and various dysrhythmias, especially tachycardia. However, in many patients abnormalities only show up on the electrocardiogram: tall right precordial R-waves, deep left precordial Q-waves or an increase of the RS ratio in the V_1. About half the patients have a low IQ (50–90). This mental retardation has been present from birth and is not progressive. It has been suggested that the increasing disability has an influence on the retardation of mental development in these children. However, the fact that children with benign infantile spinal muscular atrophy with the same severe motor handicap, and from the same social background, do not show a similar mental retardation argues against this.

In view of the far-reaching consequences of the disease for the patient and the entire family it is very important that the diagnosis is established with as much certainty as possible. The following examinations are necessary to achieve this: determination of serum creatine kinase; muscle biopsy; electromyography and electrocardiography. There is a marked rise in serum creatine kinase, with values of several thousand or tens of thousand international units found. This rise can be established soon after birth. As normal infants also show a raised serum creatine kinase until about one week after birth it is advisable to wait 2 or 3 weeks before determining its activity in infant patients with suspected Duchenne muscular dystrophy. Besides, no one can agree whether this diagnosis should be established at such an early age and the parents burdened with the knowledge. From a psychological point of view some think it better to postpone the determination of serum creatine kinase until clinical symptoms become manifest as well. It is recommended that serum creatine kinase activity is investigated in all boys of 18 months who are not yet able to walk. There are only a few neuromuscular diseases in which extremely high serum creatine kinase values are found (Table 10.1). Serum CK-MB activity is also very high without being considered a consequence of cardiomyopathy. It has been demonstrated that this MB-iso-enzyme originates in the skeletal muscles and not in the cardiac muscle. As the disease progresses serum creatine kinase decreases gradually, although it remains very high in comparison with normal values. The serum myoglobin level is always raised and some enzyme activities such as aldolase, pyruvate kinase, lactate dehydrogenase, glutamic oxaloacetic transaminase and glutamic pyruvic transaminase may also be higher. However, the rise of these enzymes is far less constant and of less diagnostic importance than the increase in serum creatine kinase.

Table 10.1. Marked increase in serum creatine kinase activity.

If a patient has a neuromuscular disease with a very high increase in serum creatine kinase (10–100 × the normal value) one should first think of:

Duchenne muscular dystrophy.
Becker muscular dystrophy.
Polymyositis and dermatomyositis.
Paroxysmal myoglobinuria (rhabdomyolysis).
Sporadic distal myopathy with early adult onset.

A biopsy is best taken from the m.quadriceps femoris as, in the ambulant patient, this muscle is ideally suited for histopathological analysis. It is important to prevent the biopsy being taken from the part of the muscle where a needle electrode, required for an electromyogram, may have been inserted earlier. Marked abnormalities have been seen in muscle biopsies of infants with Duchenne muscular dystrophy before clinical signs of the disease were demonstrated. These histopathological findings consist of marked variations in muscle fibre diameter, an increase in endomysial connective tissue and, in advanced stages, of fatty tissue as well. There are also focal abnormalities consisting of groups of necrotic and regenerating fibres and next to these, large round hyaline fibres are scattered throughout the tissue.

The electromyogram shows brief, polyphasic, low-voltage motor-unit potentials. There are never any signs of denervation and the motor and sensory conduction velocities are always normal as well. The presence of the electrocardiographic abnormalities described above strongly suggests the diagnosis, but a normal ECG does not exclude the existence of the disease.

The identification of carriers of this X-linked recessive disease plays an important role in genetic counselling. Duchenne carriers are classified as follows:

(1) Definite carriers: mothers of a son with Duchenne muscular dystrophy with another affected relative — brother, maternal uncle, nephew (on sister's side), grandson, or other male relative in the female line. Women with sons (from two different and unrelated fathers) who have Duchenne muscular dystrophy can also be viewed as definite carriers.
(2) Probable carriers: mothers with two or more sons with Duchenne muscular dystrophy who have no other male relatives in the female line with the disease.
(3) Possible carriers: mothers who have only one son with Duchenne muscular dystrophy and no other affected male relative (isolated cases; their number is estimated at about 50 per cent of the total number of cases). All other women who have a brother, a nephew (by the sister), an uncle or other male relative in the female line with Duchenne muscular dystrophy should also be viewed as possible carriers.

In a pregnant woman who is a definite carrier, four possibilities exist: she may have a son with Duchenne muscular dystrophy, she may have a healthy son, a daughter carrying Duchenne muscular dystrophy or a healthy daughter. So far there is no known method of identifying carriers with 100 per cent certainty. Until recently carrier detection depended on the estimation of the serum creatine kinase, which can be raised in carriers, usually up to twice the normal value. This determination should preferably be repeated three times at intervals of at least one week. It is also important to carry out these tests at an early age as the activity tends to decrease and sometimes return to normal in girls over 10 years of age. The value of determining creatine kinase activity in a woman who is several weeks pregnant and wants genetic advice — a situation which often occurs in practice — is made more difficult by the fact that the serum creatine kinase activity tends to decrease in early pregnancy. The neurological examination shows abnormalities in about 5 per cent of the carriers, particularly hypertrophy of the calf muscles and sometimes a slight weakness of the pelvic girdle and upper leg muscles. Other examination methods such as electromyography, electrocardiography and muscle biopsy never provide more information than the determination of serum creatine kinase. Even with this method, however, only about 80 per cent of the carriers can be detected. This means that even those women with a normal serum creatine kinase activity have about a 20 per cent chance of being a carrier after all. Recently, carriers have been detected by using a series of closely linked DNA probes detecting restriction fragment length polymorphisms (RFLPs) distributed over the short arm of the X chromosome. The ability to detect the X chromosome carrying the Duchenne muscular dystrophy gene by means of this technique is becoming increasingly successful. The technique is based on the fact that small variations in DNA formation may exist between two X chromosomes. Generally this examination requires venous blood from the patient(s) and from a number of relatives to establish whether the X chromosome with the Duchenne muscular dystrophy gene can be identified.

Carrier detection is possible if the X chromosome with the Duchenne muscular dystrophy gene and the X chromosome with the normal gene can both be identified by DNA polymorphism. Thus it can be determined, in the daughters of carriers, which of the two X chromosomes they have inherited from their mother. The reliability of this investigation increases if the identified polymorphisms are located nearer the gene involved. If the carrier is pregnant, a termination of pregnancy may be considered if a chorion villus biopsy in the 8th–10th week of pregnancy has established a male fetus; the child has a 50 per cent chance of being born with Duchenne muscular dystrophy. The 50 per cent chance that any daughter has of being a carrier must also be considered. Prenatal diagnosis of the disease based on serum creatine kinase determinations in fetal blood has been described, but such methods are still in the research stage and cannot be considered routine. In some cases prenatal diagnosis is also possible by using closely linked RFLPs.

No drug is known to halt or even improve the disease process. On the other hand, close support (also of the parents!), regular monitoring, and long-term physiotherapy, as well as orthopaedic aids are all important for the patient's well-being and quality of life. Physiotherapy should first concentrate on controlling the flexion contractures of the hips and feet. The patient walks on his toes in order to keep his balance, and improvement of the pes equinus by means of surgery will actually make walking worse for him. Stretching the Achilles tendons and night splints are especially successful in young children. Although they continue to walk on their toes, standing becomes easier.

There are no agreed surgical guidelines, but there are basically two approaches: one aims to keep the patient on his feet for as long as possible by surgical means (lengthening of the Achilles tendons, moving the tendon of the m.tibialis posterior, cutting the tendon of the m.tensor fascia lata); the other attempts to avoid surgery as much as possible and accepts the disadvantage of the patient requiring a wheelchair at an earlier stage. In the end, the patient proves to be considerably more mobile in his electric wheelchair than either he or his parents would have thought and a great deal of time and effort can now be devoted to leisure and hobbies instead of post-operative care and orthopaedic aids. It is known that surgery may worsen the patient's condition and that patients who were able to walk before the operation may no longer do so afterwards. Everybody will know of an example of the catastrophic results of such a 'successful' operation for the patient. Nevertheless, it is apparent that very good results can be obtained with the right indication and experience, and after carefully choosing the time of surgery, together with expert pre- and post-operative physiotherapy and modern long leg braces of light-weight material.

Postscript

Observing how a child walks and stands is more important for the diagnosis of Duchenne muscular dystrophy than a neurological examination.

The best way to diagnose the disease is to listen carefully to the mother.

Duchenne muscular dystrophy is in fact a congenital myopathy which can be diagnosed soon after birth by means of a muscle biopsy and determination of serum creatine kinase activity.

In a young boy with extremely high serum creatine kinase activity one should think firstly of Duchenne muscular dystrophy, secondly of Duchenne muscular dystrophy, and finally of Duchenne muscular dystrophy.

In the case of a young boy who was late in learning to walk, who falls frequently and has flat feet, the last thing one should think of is arch supports.

The only one pleased with a surgical correction of the equinus position of the feet in a young Duchenne muscular dystrophy patient is the surgeon himself.

When diagnosing Duchenne muscular dystrophy one should always remember the patient's sisters; after all, they may be carriers of the gene for this disease.

11

Becker-type muscular dystrophy

In many ways Becker-type muscular dystrophy (BMD) can be considered a benign form of Duchenne muscular dystrophy. The gene for BMD is also located at the short arm of the X chromosome. For that reason the disease is also called benign X-linked muscular dystrophy. There are no reliable data as to its prevalence and incidence. The age of onset can vary from the first years of life to the late thirties. The average age at which the first signs appear is about 10–11 years. Although the initial stages of the disease can resemble Duchenne muscular dystrophy, in 90 per cent of patients with Becker muscular dystrophy the first signs appear after the fifth year of life. Although its course is always progressive, the speed of progression is extremely varied, even within families.

The first symptoms often consist of muscle cramps after exercise, especially in the calf muscles. This complaint is rarely voiced spontaneously, but with prompting, 90 per cent of patients reveal that they have regular muscle cramps. In the early stages of the disease patients also complain of falling frequently and of having difficulty in running and climbing stairs, while there is often a tendency to walk on tip-toe as well. Examination will show a weakness of the pelvic girdle and upper leg muscles, with the m.gluteus maximus being particularly affected. Usually there is also weakness of the shoulder girdle and upper arm muscles, although to a lesser extent, thus creating the typical picture of a limb-girdle syndrome. The neck flexors are regularly involved as is the distal musculature, though the latter only slightly, leaving the small muscles of the hand always unaffected. In general, the upper leg extensors are more affected than the flexors.

Besides atrophy (especially of the upper leg musculature), hypertrophy of the calf muscles is found in about 80 per cent of patients with BMD (Fig. 11.1). Although contractures of the ankles and hips develop in about half the patients, shortening of other muscles (m.rectus femoris, m.pectoralis major, the hamstrings) play a modest role. It is important that the occurrence of pes equinus does not correlate with the duration of the disease. On the other hand there seems to be a clear correlation between the duration of the illness and the disappearance of the myotatic reflexes: the knee jerks are the first to become negative, followed by the reflexes of the arm and, in the final stage, the ankle jerks.

Cardiac abnormalities are found in about 50 per cent of patients. This cardiomyopathy rarely manifests itself clinically and cardiac auscultation and radiography of the thorax will not provide relevant information about the condition of the cardiac muscle either. Electrocardiography and echocardiography are the most useful methods of demonstrating cardiomyopathy. The ECG shows the same abnormalities as in Duchenne muscular dystrophy: deep in left precordial Q-waves, ST-segment changes and/or an increase in the RS ratio in V_1. Echocardiography may identify dilatation of the left ventricle, as well as reduced excursion of the

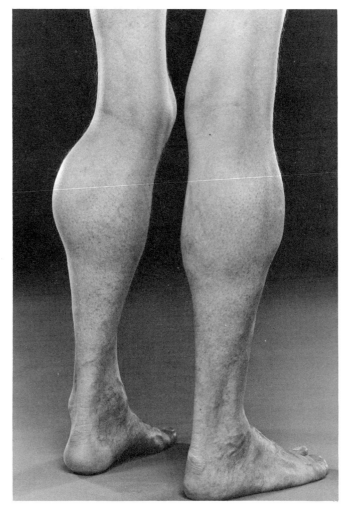

Fig. 11.1. Becker-type muscular dystrophy. Hypertrophy of the calf muscles. Computed tomography of these muscles revealed that large parts of the muscle tissue had been replaced by fatty tissue. This makes it a pseudohypertrophy.

posterior wall of the left ventricle and of the interventricular septum. The fact that the involvement of the cardiac muscle in BMD does not depend on the patient's age, disease duration and/

or the degree of weakness of the skeletal muscles is important for practical reasons. Thus, young patients, who only suffer slight weakness for a short time, may nevertheless show clear abnormalities on the ECG.

Serum creatine kinase activity is at least five times and sometimes as much as 100 or more times as high as normal values. Activity is very high in young patients who have not had the disease long, but decreases with age and disease duration. Serum CK-MB activity is also markedly increased and is not related to the presence of cardiomyopathy. As in Duchenne muscular dystrophy, it is assumed that the MB-iso-enzyme is produced by the skeletal muscle rather than the cardiac muscle. Electromyography shows not only brief, low-voltage action potentials but also spontaneous fibrillation, positive denervation potentials and high-voltage polyphasic action potentials. A predominance of type-1 fibres is found in about 50 per cent of muscle biopsies. There is also a marked variation in fibre diameter and an increase in the number of fibres with internal nuclei. As in Duchenne muscular dystrophy there are swollen hyaline fibres scattered throughout the tissue, and groups of necrotic and regenerating fibres. Later, however, changes associated with chronic denervation are seen as well, including small groups of small angular fibres as well as clusters of hyperchromatic and pyknotic nuclei. Computed tomography of the muscles involved reveals low-density areas corresponding to the density of fatty tissues. At the beginning, these areas are only observed in parts of the muscle, but eventually the entire muscle is replaced by fatty tissue, the fascia remaining visible for a long time. In addition, one can often observe a hypertrophy of the medial head of the m.gastrocnemius, the m.sartorius, the m.gracilis and the m.adductor longus.

At first the genes responsible for Becker and Duchenne muscular dystrophies were thought to be alleles; then it was discovered that the loci of the genes of both these diseases were a considerable distance from each other. This meant that the two conditions were not different expressions of the same gene, but that they involved different genes. The possibilities of identifying carriers with the BMD gene are very limited indeed: only about 50 per cent of the definite carriers appear to have an increased serum creatine kinase activity. There are indications that carrier detection with closely linked restriction fragment length polymorphisms (page 71) will give more reliable results. All daughters of a BMD patient are definite carriers because they always inherit one X chromosome carrying the abnormal gene from the father. A differential diagnosis with Duchenne muscular dystrophy will only present difficulties with the very small group of Becker-type muscular dystrophy patients who show signs at a very young age and who have no other relatives in the maternal line with this disease (isolated cases). In such cases it is mainly the course of the disease which determines the diagnosis. Emery and Skinner demonstrated that 96.9 per cent of patients with BMD did not need a wheelchair before the age of 11.2 years (mean age 27). By contrast, the same percentage of patients with Duchenne muscular dystrophy are no longer able to walk at the age of 11.2 years (mean age 8.6 years).

Physiotherapy may be considered although excessive exercise of the muscles must be avoided, particularly as many patients then complain of muscle cramps. The treatment of contractures should remain conservative for as long as possible.

12

Facioscapulohumeral dystrophy

Facioscapulohumeral dystrophy, or Landouzy–Déjérine disease, is an autosomal dominant and slowly progressive disease whose expression is markedly variable. The age of onset is often difficult to establish; it may begin in childhood and yet sometimes only becomes manifest in adult life. Generally, however, the first symptoms and signs occur in the teenage years. The disease often commences with bilateral and often asymmetric involvement of the facial muscles. Consequently, most patients report that they cannot whistle. The patient's history may reveal that he was unable to drink lemonade with a straw or blow up a balloon when a child. His parents may also report that his eyes are never entirely closed during sleep.

On inspection the patient's face shows poor expression with almost no wrinkles on the forehead. Ptosis, as seen in dystrophia myotonica (see Fig. 19.1) hardly ever occurs with this condition. If the patient is asked to close the eyes very tightly then the lashes will remain visible (Fig. 12.1). It is impossible for the patient to purse his lips or whistle, and he has difficulty puffing out his cheeks. When smiling, the corners of the mouth are pulled laterally. Sometimes there is an abnormal protrusion of the upper lip ('bouche de tapir'), but this phenomenon, although often described in the literature, is in fact very rare. Dysarthria may develop if the facial muscles are severely affected.

Most patients are only bothered by the disease once the shoulder girdle muscles weaken. Facioscapulohumeral dystrophy is a disease which is often markedly asymmetric in an early stage. Thus, a weakness of the shoulder girdle muscles may, for years, be only manifest on one side. Primarily, there is a difficulty in elevating the arms to above shoulder height experienced, for example, when lifting heavy objects or combing the hair. The lower and middle parts of the m.trapezius, the m.serratus anterior, the m.latissimus dorsi, the m.rhomboideus and the m.pectoralis major (particularly the sternal part) are affected first. The fact that the m.deltoideus is hardly weakened, if at all, is noteworthy. Therefore, the inability to raise the arms is not the result of weakness of the deltoid muscles, as is often incorrectly assumed, but is instead only due to the fact that the scapulae cannot be fixed. Asking the patient to stretch his arms before him or to abduct them will give rise to scapulae alatae with a very prominent angulus inferior and a lateral elevation of the scapulae (Figs. 12.2 and 12.3). Inspecting the patient from the front, the upper parts of the scapulae are seen to protrude in a place where one would normally observe the trapezius muscles. The neck flexors, especially the sternal part of the mm.sternocleidomastoidei may also be weakened. In the upper arms the m.biceps and the m.brachioradialis are usually involved earlier and also to a greater extent than the m.triceps.

The process, however, does not stop at facioscapulohumeral muscle weakness. Many other muscles may weaken as well, sometimes at an early stage in the disease. This has been demonstrated by means of computed tomography. The abdominal muscles, the hamstrings, the m.tibialis anterior, the m.extensor

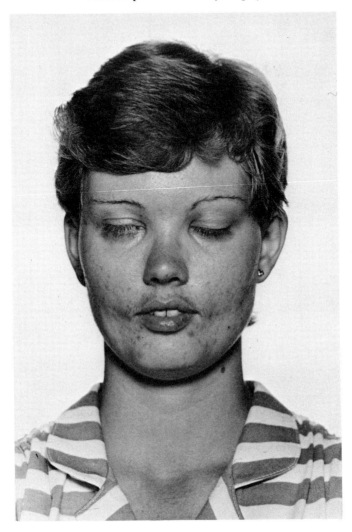

Fig. 12.1. Facioscapulohumeral dystrophy. With maximal contraction of the orbicularis oculi muscles the eyelashes remain visible. There is a positive Bell's phenomenon in the right eye.

hallucis longus and the medial head of the m.gastrocnemius appear to be involved at an early stage. The m.quadriceps and the m.peroneus, however, appear to remain unaffected for a long

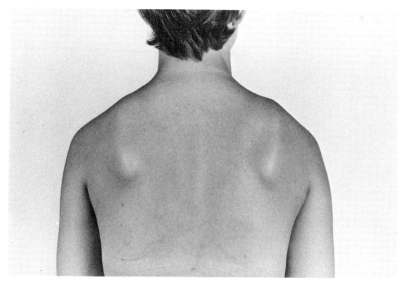

Fig. 12.2. Facioscapulohumeral dystrophy. At rest the shoulders are in anteposition and hang down. There is a slight winging and some lateral deviation of the scapulae.

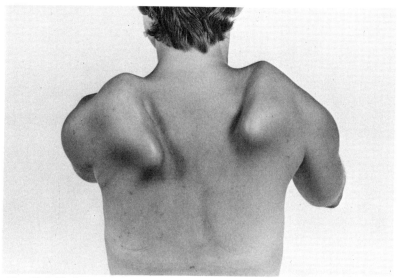

Fig. 12.3. Facioscapulohumeral dystrophy. When the arms are raised, the winging of the scapulae is accentuated, while there is also an elevation of the scapulae.

time. The myotatic reflexes of the arms are usually poor or absent, the knee jerks may be impaired, but the ankle jerks remain normal for a long time. Serum creatine kinase activity may be normal or slightly increased, especially in young patients. Electromyography reveals the presence of brief polyphasic action potentials with a low amplitude. These supplementary examinations do not contribute to the diagnosis, nor does a muscle biopsy. Apart from a marked variability in muscle-fibre diameter, small groups of angular fibres can sometimes be observed, and this is suggestive of a neurogenic factor. Additionally, lobulated type-1 fibres (motheaten fibres) may be present. Finally, cell infiltrates consisting of lymphocytes and sometimes plasma cells are also often seen. Once, patients with such cell infiltrates in their muscle biopsies were recommended for treatment with corticosteroids, but it is now generally recognized that this therapy does not have any effect on the course of the disease. Cardiac muscle is not involved in this disease.

The disease usually has a benign course; thus, patients can remain ambulant for as many as 40 years, and perhaps for the rest of their lives.

Many authors indicate that abortive cases occur frequently with the patient showing, for example, only a slight weakness of the facial muscles or an abnormal position of one or both shoulders. Approximately 30 per cent of the patients have no complaints. In some patients, however, most of the muscles of the trunk and limbs are involved and this results in very serious disability. The seriousness of the disease not only varies widely between families but also within families as well. This means that a patient who is only slightly affected can have a child in whom the disease can develop severely (and vice versa). This must be taken into account in genetic counselling. Ankle-foot athrodeses are suitable for those patients who have a considerable weakness of the m.tibialis anterior. Arm elevation can be increased considerably if the scapula is fixed to the thoracic wall, which would improve the function of the intact m.deltoideus. Several surgical techniques have been recommended for this.

In a patient with a facioscapulohumeral syndrome (Table 12.1) one should first think of Landouzy–Déjérine disease. This diagnosis can only be given with certainty after an autosomal dominant mode of inheritance has been demonstrated. Because of

Table 12.1. The facioscapulohumeral syndrome.

Facioscapulohumeral dystrophy (Landouzy–Déjérine disease).
Infantile facioscapulohumeral dystrophy.
Facioscapulohumeral spinal muscular atrophy.
Myopathy with abnormal mitochondria.

The syndome occurs less frequently and/or in a less pure form in:
Central core disease.
Nemaline myopathy (rod disease).
Myotubular myopathy.
Polymyositis.
Myasthenia gravis.

---

the high incidence of abortive cases it is absolutely necessary to include an examination of the family (parents!). Sporadic and autosomal recessive cases have also been described; these are often very progressive, similar to the infantile form which occurs in the first years of life. Weakness of the facial musculature may be absent in some patients with Landouzy–Déjérine disease. If a patient with weakness of the shoulder-girdle muscles has simultaneous weakness of the foot flexors, he is considered to have a scapuloperoneal syndrome (see Table 12.1).

13

The scapuloperoneal syndrome

The combination of a weakness of the shoulder-girdle muscles and a weakness of the m.tibialis anterior and mm.peronei is characteristic of the scapuloperoneal syndrome. This combination of muscle weaknesses may occur in numerous myogenic and neurogenic conditions (Table 13.1). The pure scapuloperoneal syndrome, on the other hand, is rare; as a rule other muscle groups are also

Table 13.1. The scapuloperoneal syndrome.

Muscle is site of primary lesion.
Scapuloperoneal myopathy:
— sporadic.
— autosomal dominant.
— X-linked recessive.*
Facioscapulohumeral dystrophy (variable expressivity of gene).

Anterior horn cell is site of primary lesion.
Scapuloperoneal spinal muscular atrophy.
— sporadic.
— autosomal dominant.
— X-linked recessive.

Peripheral nerve is site of primary lesion.
Scapuloperoneal atrophy
With sensory abnormalities (Davidenkov syndrome):
— sporadic.
— autosomal dominant.
— autosomal recessive.
Without sensory abnormalities:
— sporadic.

Myogenic and neurogenic lesions are both present.
— sporadic.
— autosomal dominant.
— X-linked recessive.

---

*Some of these diseases are associated with cardiomyopathy.

affected, to a greater or lesser degree, as for example, the facial musculature, the neck extensors or pelvic girdle muscles.

Autosomal dominant scapuloperoneal myopathy

This may begin in childhood, usually with a weakness of the foot extensors. These muscles gradually become wasted, so that in the beginning the picture may well be confused with a hereditary motor and sensory neuropathy. In the latter, however, the m.extensor digitorum brevis is atrophic while it remains intact or is often hypertrophic in scapuloperoneal myopathy because the patient continues to contract it in an effort at dorsiflexion of the foot. The condition usually progresses very slowly. As in so many autosomal dominant diseases there may be a strong variability in gene expression: the onset may not occur until adulthood, the first signs may become manifest in the shoulder-girdle muscles, while the speed of progression can also be very different, not only between families but within them as well. The reflexes of the biceps, the triceps and the ankles are usually poor or absent. Serum creatine kinase activity is generally normal or only slightly increased. Weakness of the facial musculature may occur in many patients and, if it does, differentiation from facioscapulohumeral muscular dystrophy becomes difficult since, in the latter disease, the lower-leg extensors are often affected as well. Consequently, many authors believe that scapuloperoneal myopathy should be considered a variant of facioscapulohumeral muscular dystrophy.

X-linked recessive scapuloperoneal syndrome

This has been described under different names, including scapulo-humerodistal muscular dystrophy, scapuloperoneal atrophy, and humeroperoneal neuromuscular disease. The onset occurs in childhood, usually before the age of 10. The first symptoms consist in shortening and contracture of the calf muscles (pes equinus), the m.biceps (flexion contractures of the elbows) and the paravertebral muscles (rigid spine syndrome). The patients experience difficulty in flexing the neck and in bending forward. Besides scapuloperoneal muscle weakness and wasting, a cardiomyopathy appears to occur in many patients as well. Owing to an associated atrioventricular block many patients may die suddenly, the average age being 45.

Although some authors include the Emery–Dreyfuss type of muscular dystrophy as a scapuloperoneal syndrome, an X-linked recessive limb-girdle syndrome is always present here. On the other hand, flexion contractures of the elbows, contractures of the Achilles tendons and sometimes also a cardiomyopathy can develop in this disease, even in childhood.

Postscript

The scapuloperoneal syndrome rarely occurs in its pure form.

Autosomal dominant scapuloperoneal myopathy is probably a variant of autosomal dominant facioscapulohumeral dystrophy. Given that the scapuloperoneal syndrome can be caused by a lesion of the muscles, the peripheral nerves, the anterior horn cells, or any combination of these, and that its inheritance can be autosomal recessive, dominant, X-linked or can even be non-hereditary, it is obvious that it is a condition capable of causing great confusion.

The confusion starts with the name: on the one hand a bone (the scapula) is mentioned and on the other hand a nerve (the n.peroneus), while the aim is to indicate the extent of the muscle weakness.

14

The limb-girdle syndrome

Limb-girdle muscular dystrophy has been known in myology for over 30 years. It refers to a form of muscular dystrophy which mostly or exclusively involves the muscles of the shoulder and pelvic girdles as well as the proximal muscles of the limbs. The name was first used in 1953 by Stevenson who subdivided all muscular dystrophies into Duchenne disease and autosomal limb-girdle muscular dystrophy. One year later, Walton and Nattrass distinguished three different diseases — exclusively on clinical grounds — namely, Duchenne's disease, facioscapulohumeral muscular dystrophy and limb-girdle muscular dystrophy. Limb-girdle muscular dystrophy usually begins between the tenth and thirtieth year, although sometimes in middle age too. The mode of inheritance of the disease is usually recessive; the autosomal dominant form is rare. The first signs consist of weakness in the muscles of the shoulder or pelvic girdle. The speed of progression is variable: fast in some patients and slow in others; it usually leads to serious disability and reduces life expectancy.

This type of variable symptomatology could apply to many diseases. Nor has this clinical picture become more uniform over the years. There is insufficient information about whether or not there are muscle contractures and muscular atrophy. Serum creatine kinase activity is sometimes slightly and sometimes moderately increased. The electromyogram shows brief action potentials of low amplitude and an increase in the number of polyphasic potentials. On its own, however, this finding is of limited diagnostic value since it occurs in many myogenic and chronic neurogenic disorders. A variety of muscle biopsy abnormalities have been described. Some authors attach considerable

Table 14.1. Neuromuscular diseases presenting with a limb-girdle syndrome.

Benign infantile (or juvenile) spinal muscular atrophy.
Polymyositis and dermatomyositis.
Duchenne muscular dystrophy.
Becker-type muscular dystrophy.

Congenital myopathy with contractures.
Emery–Dreifuss dystrophy.
Acid maltase deficiency.
Myophosphorylase deficiency.
Muscle carnitine deficiency.
Central core disease.
Nemaline myopathy (rod disease).
Myopathies with abnormal mitochondria.
Carcinoid myopathy.
Thyrotoxic myopathy.
Myopathy in hyperparathyroidism.
Myopathy in acromegaly.
Myopathy in Cushing syndrome.
Myopathy in hyperaldosteronism.
Familial periodic paralyses (during attack or persistent).
Alcoholic myopathy.
Corticosteroid myopathy.
Chloroquine myopathy.

In the differential diagnosis of a limb-girdle syndrome, the first four diseases mentioned in this table should be considered first.

diagnostic importance to the presence of hypertrophic or split muscle fibres, or to a substantial increase in endomysial connective tissue. Others, however, conclude the opposite, or suggest that myogenic and neurogenic disorders always occur together. The fact remains that there is no uniform description of the abnormalities found in muscle biopsies of limb-girdle muscular dystrophy patients.

Consequently, it is not surprising that a clear clinical picture of limb-girdle muscular dystrophy proves impossible, because each author's description differs and simply quotes the old clinical observations of the past. As more and improved diagnostic techniques become available, so the diagnosis of limb-girdle muscular dystrophy appears to be made less often. Consequently, it is our opinion that limb-girdle muscular dystrophy does not exist and that we should speak of a limb-girdle syndrome instead. It is generally assumed that many patients who were earlier considered to have limb-girdle muscular dystrophy really suffered from benign infantile spinal muscular atrophy (Wohlfart–Kugelberg–Welander disease). In addition, there are many other neuromuscular diseases in which the syndrome occurs (Table 14.1). The syndrome may only occur during a certain stage of these diseases. It is often the first stage in serious progressive diseases, but may last much longer in chronic and slowly progressive diseases.

15

Distal myopathies

There is a rule of thumb in myology which says that distal weakness is associated with neurogenic disorders, while in myogenic disorders the proximal muscles are the first to be affected. There are myopathies, though, which predominantly or exclusively affect the distal musculature. Nevertheless, it remains the correct procedure to think first of a neurogenic cause in patients with a distal weakness (Table 15.1). In addition to this,

Table 15.1. Neuromuscular diseases presenting with mainly distal muscular weakness.

Polyneuropathies.
Hereditary motor and sensory neuropathies.
Amyotrophic lateral sclerosis.
Distal spinal muscular atrophy.
Myotonic dystrophy.
Scapuloperoneal syndrome.
Congenital distal myopathy.
Infantile distal myopathy.
Late onset distal myopathy.
Sporadic distal myopathy with early adult onset.
Myopathia distalis tarda hereditaria (Welander disease).
Distal myopathy with abnormal mitochondria.
Distal polymyositis.
Inclusion body myositis.

---

most distal myopathies show signs that the peripheral motor neuron is affected as well. The majority of distal myopathies are autosomal dominant, although autosomal recessive and so-called sporadic cases occur as well. The condition can be congenital or it may develop in infancy or in adult life.

Congenital and infantile distal myopathies

These myopathies are extremely rare: only a few patients and families have been described. The symptoms generally begin in the muscles of the lower legs and feet and are sometimes followed by weakness of the distal muscles of the upper limbs. Abnormal mitochondria have been found in the muscle fibres of some patients and because of this these conditions can be included in the group of congenital myopathies with abnormal mitochondria.

Myopathia distalis tarda hereditaria

This is an autosomal dominant condition which occurs in Sweden. Most patients described in other countries have proved to be of Swedish origin. The disease was first recognized by Welander

(1951) who, in her thesis, gave a detailed description of the signs shown by 249 patients from 72 different families.

The first complaints appear around the age of 50 and usually consist of cold hands and difficulty with fine movements of the fingers (doing up buttons, taking money from a wallet). The signs often begin in one thumb and/or index finger. Gradually, weakness and wasting of the lower arm extensors and the small muscles of the hands develop. Finally, the lower leg extensors become involved as well. At this time the ankle jerk may also disappear; the other myotatic reflexes remain intact.

Sporadic distal myopathy with early adult onset

This is a slowly progressive condition in which the first signs occur in the legs. Sometimes the calf muscles are especially weakened and wasted and, if this is the case, the patient will still be able to walk on his heels, but not on his toes. This type of finding is rare in neuromuscular disease: usually patients are able to walk on their toes, but not their heels. Gradually the extensors of the lower leg become weak as well and, finally, the lower arm and hand muscles. Yet slight signs of involvement of the proximal muscles of the legs are often found in this distal myopathy. Computed tomography regularly shows, among other things, low densities in the m.gluteus minimus on both sides. Both knee and ankle jerk reflexes are usually absent.

A markedly large increase in serum creatine kinase activity (up to more than 30 times the normal value) is very characteristic for this disease. Apart from brief, low-voltage and polyphasic potentials, electromyograms also show fibrillations and positive sharp waves. The motor and sensory nerve conduction velocities are normal. The muscle biopsy shows degeneration and regeneration as well as vacuoles, too many fibres with internal nuceli, and small groups of small angular fibres. Thus, both electromyography and histopathology show not only myogenic abnormalities but also abnormalities which could fit a neurogenic disorder.

16

Progressive external ophthalmoplegia

The eye muscles are a special type of skeletal muscle. Clinically, we can examine their function but not their strength. They do not tire very easily. There are only three to ten muscle fibres per motor unit. Apart from a low innervation ratio there is a high neuron firing rate. The normal action potentials in the eye muscles are very brief. For that reason the interpretation of electromyograms of the extraocular muscles is very difficult and requires great experience. There are marked differences in architecture, innervation, morphology, and histochemical properties between the eye muscles and other skeletal muscles. The m.obliquus inferior is usually the preferred muscle for biopsy. There are a wide range of often rare diseases which cause a slowly progressive weakness of the extraocular muscles (Table 16.1). This chapter will discuss those conditions which are usually included in the group of ocular myopathies.

Ocular myopathy

The onset of ocular myopathy can be at any age but is usually between 20 and 30. The first sign is usually ptosis; thus the patient is inclined to tilt his head backwards and wrinkle his forehead to compensate. The involvement of the extraocular muscles occurs so insidiously and the progression of the weakness is so slow that the patient never complains of double vision. After many years the facial musculature may also become involved, followed by weakness of the neck, trunk, and upper arm muscles. Serum creatine kinase activity may be increased slightly to moderately.

It is very likely that the condition is a syndrome rather than a disease in itself. This is suggested by the fact that both autosomal recessive and dominant forms exist. Sporadic cases have also been described and some patients have shown an abnormal sensitivity to curare. It is quite possible that many of the patients thought to have ocular myopathy in the past would now be diagnosed as having oculocraniosomatic neuromuscular disease.

Table 16.1. Diseases which may be associated with progressive external ophthalmoplegia.

Ocular myopathy.
Oculopharyngeal myopathy.
Oculocraniosomatic neuromuscular disease (Kearns–Sayre syndrome).
Mitochondrial encephalomyopathies.
Myotubular myopathy.
Centronuclear myopathy.
Focal loss of cross-striations.
Multicore disease.
Myotonic dystrophy.
Polymyositis (rare).
Ocular myositis.
Carnitine deficiency.
Myasthenia gravis.
Ocular myopathy with abnormal sensitivity to curare.
Neuropathies (diabetes mellitus; Miller–Fisher syndrome).
Ophthalmopathy in Graves' disease (dysthyroid ophthalmopathy).
Progressive juvenile bulbar palsy (Fazio–Londe disease).
Chronic vitamin-E deficiency (in cystic fibrosis).
Nuclear and supranuclear conditions (often with other systemic degenerations).

Oculopharyngeal myopathy

This disease is associated with a slowly progressive ptosis and dysphagia. Usually it does not begin before 40 to 50 years of age. Sometimes there may be slight involvement of the facial muscles. In spite of its name the extraocular muscles become involved at a very late stage, if at all, with the exception of the m.levator palpebrae. The majority of patients described come from one French-Canadian family in which the disease appeared to be autosomal dominant. The literature reports other patients who have ptosis and dysphagia, sometimes associated with mild involvement of the muscles of the shoulder and pelvic girdle and the distal muscles of the legs.

Oculocraniosomatic neuromuscular disease

In 1958, Kearns and Sayre described a syndrome consisting of external ophthalmoplegia, pigment degeneration of the retina and complete heart block. In subsequent years it became clear that these three symptoms formed part of oculocraniosomatic neuromuscular disease, also named ophthalmoplegia plus, Kearns–Sayre syndrome or Kearns–Shy syndrome.

The disease can occur at any age, although it usually begins in late childhood or puberty. There is bilateral ptosis and weakness of the extraocular muscles, but the patients do not complain of diplopia. Sometimes there is also some weakness of the facial muscles. Weakness of the neck muscles, the proximal and/or distal muscles of the limbs or of the shoulder and pelvic girdle musculature is observed in about half the patients. Early onset is usually associated with mental retardation and retarded growth. As a rule the CSF protein level is raised. Cerebellar ataxia and neural deafness may also occur. Many patients also have endocrine disorders such as pituitary dysfunction, delayed puberty, amenorrhoea, diabetes mellitus, hypoparathyroidism, and hyperaldosteronism.

Neuropathological findings in the brain include vacuolation of the white matter and several nuclei (globus pallidus, red nucleus, vestibular nuclei). This spongiform encephalopathy can also be demonstrated with computed tomography. The final aid to the diagnosis is the finding of muscle fibres with abnormal mitochondria (ragged red fibres, see p. 103) in the muscle biopsy. These fibres occur also in the muscles of patients in whom the examination did not show any muscle weakness. The number of these abnormal fibres may fluctuate from 1–25 per cent; there is no correlation between the number of ragged red fibres and the duration of the disease. Abnormal mitochondria can be observed not only in the muscle fibres, but also in the cerebellum, the liver and the sweat glands. No therapy is available for this multisystemic condition. Pacemaker implantation may be indicated if the heart muscle shows severe conduction disturbances.

17

Congenital myopathies

The congenital myopathies form a group of diseases which are usually hereditary and not, or only very slowly, progressive. They are nearly always named after the histopathologic findings in the muscle biopsy (Table 17.1). In addition, there are a number of congenital myogenic conditions which are not included in the congenital myopathies in a narrower sense, usually for clinical reasons (Table 17.1). Finally, there are also diseases which can be identified immediately after birth by biochemical examination, although the clinical signs will only become manifest after several months: Duchenne muscular dystrophy and infantile acid-maltase deficiency (Pompe's disease).

The clinical pictures of most congenital myopathies are nearly identical. Signs that the child suffers from a myopathy are sometimes already present before birth: the mother often mentions that she has noticed reduced fetal movements during pregnancy. The fetus has difficulty in swallowing in some congenital myopathies, which may give rise to a hydramnios in the last months of pregnancy. These signs are also known to occur in congenital myotonic dystrophy (see p. 116). The children show a marked generalized hypotonia (floppy babies) immediately following birth. Weakness of the muscles is also apparent; as a rule the pelvic girdle and upper leg muscles are more often affected than the shoulder girdle and upper arm muscles. However, a generalized muscle weakness also occurs. The muscles are often underdeveloped. Often this has been called 'atrophy' of the musculature, although strictly speaking atrophy means that the muscle was normal before it began to decrease in bulk. In children with a congenital myopathy, however, markedly thin arms and legs are seen immediately after birth. Thus, we should speak of muscle hypotrophy instead. In some congenital myopathies there is weakness of the facial and/or extraocular muscles (Table 17.2, Figs. 17.1–17.4). It is of practical importance to know that patients with eye-muscle weakness never complain of double vision. The skull is often long and narrow with a high arched palate. Other

93

Table 17.1. Congenital neuromuscular diseases.

Congenital myopathies.
Cap disease.
Central core disease.
Centronuclear myopathy.
Congenital fibre-type disproportion.
Congenital lipid-storage disease.
Congenital mitochondria–lipid–glycogen disease.
Fingerprint body myopathy.
Focal loss of cross-striations.
Minicore disease.
Multicore disease.
Myopathy with lysis of myofibrils.
Myopathy with bodies containing sulphydryl groups.
Myotubular myopathy.
Nemaline myopathy (rod disease).
Reducing body myopathy.
Sarcotubular myopathy.
Type-1-fibre atrophy and myotube-like structures.
Type-1-fibre hypoplasia and myasthenic features.
Type-1-fibre hypotrophy with central nuclei.

Other congenital neuromuscular diseases.
Congenital cerebromuscular dystrophy (Fukuyama).
Congenital distal myopathy.
Congenital myotonic dystrophy.
Congenital myopathy with abnormal mitochondria.
Congenital myopathy with contractures (Bethlem–van Wijngaarden).
Congenital phosphofructokinase deficiency.
Myotonia congenita:
— autosomal dominant type (Thomsen).
— autosomal recessive type (Becker).
Congenital hereditarry motor and sensory neuropathy.
Congenital myasthenia.
Infantile spinal muscular atrophy (Werdnig–Hoffmann disease).

The diseases known as congenital myopathies show almost identical clinical features. Other congenital neuromuscular diseases have, as a rule, a different clinical picture.

skeletal changes such as hip dislocation, pes cavus, or kyphoscoliosis are also fairly frequent.

In general, motor development is slow: children are late sitting, standing and walking. They fall down often when walking and they are never able to run. They are poor at gymnastics: skipping and vaulting prove impossible. They cannot pull themselves up on rings or horizontal bars. They will be the last to be chosen for team games and they will usually be goalkeeper in soccer. The

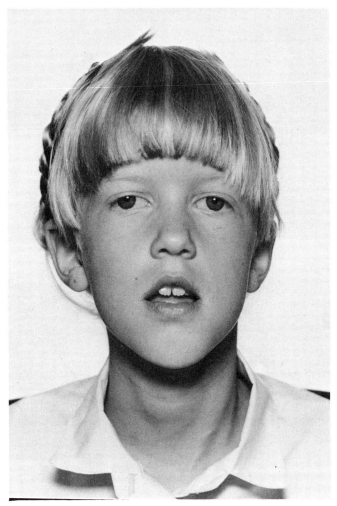

Fig. 17.1. Congenital myopathy (focal loss of cross-striations). There is a bilateral facial weakness. The face is elongated, the upper lip is tented and the mouth is kept open.

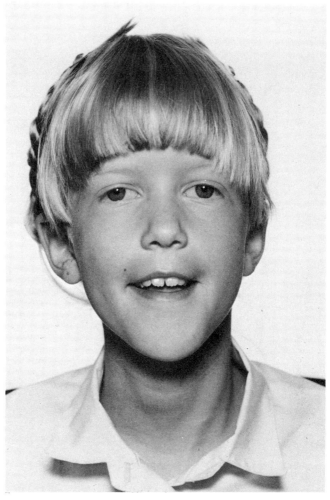

Fig. 17.2. Congenital myopathy. When laughing, the corners of the mouth are mostly pulled laterally.

inevitable teasing and frustration associated with this are responsible for the fact that in later life these children — who almost always have normal or good intelligence — indicate that they were never very interested in sports.

The reflexes are normal, low or absent. Serum creatine kinase

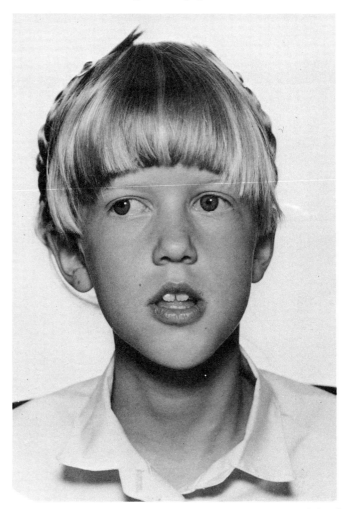

Fig. 17.3. Congenital myopathy. Apart from involvement of the facial muscles the extraocular muscles are also weakened. In an attempt to look as far as possible to the right, horizontal eye movements appear to be restricted.

activity is normal or sometimes slightly increased. The electromyogram shows short-duration, small-amplitude, and polyphasic motor potentials. The motor and sensory conduction velocities are normal.

The fact that the muscle weakness is not, or is only very slowly, progressive in many of the congenital myopathies is important. This means that the parents can be given a clear picture of the child's future possibilities at an early stage. There is little point in prescribing long-term muscle-strengthening exercises to these

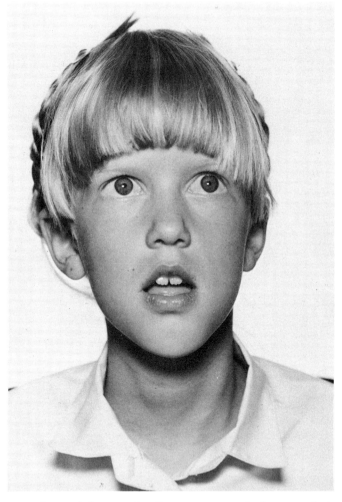

Fig. 17.4. Congenital myopathy. In an attempt to look up, vertical eye movements appear to have become virtually impossible.

Table 17.2 Congenital myopathies associated with weakness of the facial (F) and/or extraocular (EO) muscles.

Disease	F	EO
Cap disease.	+	−
Central core disease.	+	−
Centronuclear myopathy.	−	+
Congenital fibre-type disproportionate	+	−
Focal loss of cross-striations	−	+
Myotubular myopathy	+	+
Minicore disease	+	−
Multicore disease	+	+
Myopathy with lysis of myofibrils	+	+
Nemaline myopathy (rod disease)	+	−
Reducing body myopathy	+	+
Sarcotubular myopathy	+	−

patients. Physiotherapy is only indicated if there is a tendency to develop contractures, although this only occurs in a minority of cases.

The congenital myopathies cannot be classified on the basis of the clinical picture (which is almost identical for each form). The cause of this group of diseases is unknown, which makes a classification based on aetiology impossible.

A classification on the basis of mode of inheritance is not helpful either. This was the reason why the different diseases had to be named after the histopathologic findings in the muscle biopsy. It is remarkable that type-1 fibres predominate in nearly all congenital myopathies (type-1-fibre predominance). Some of the most frequent congenital myopathies are discussed below, emphasis being given to histopathologic changes.

Central core disease

Both autosomal dominant and non-hereditary (sporadic) forms of this disease have been described. Congenital hip dislocation is found relatively often. The clinical picture shows a marked variation: patients without or with very few complaints of muscle weakness have been described. If there is muscle weakness it is not progressive. Patients with central core disease have an increased risk of developing malignant hyperthermia during general anaesthesia. This is of practical importance in these patients because they are often operated upon for pes equinus or hip dislocation.

In the muscle biopsy, apart from type-1-fibre predominance, collections of abnormal myofibrils in the muscle fibres (mostly type-1 fibres) are observed. These abnormal fibrils or 'cores' are often located in the centre of the fibre, although they can occur in the periphery too. Most fibres contain only one core, although more — up to 5 per fibre — may occur. Electron microscopy reveals that there are no mitochondria in these cores. Consequently, the cores — which can be observed along the entire length of the muscle fibre — do not show any mitochondria-associated oxidative enzyme activity.

Nemaline myopathy (rod disease)

There is both an autosomal recessive and an autosomal dominant form of this condition. Apart from a dolichocephalic skull, many paients also have an elongated face, a high arched palate, and an underdeveloped ('hypotrophic') musculature. Apart from a generalized weakness, there is often a facial weakness. The muscle weakness is progressive in about half the patients. Serious signs may sometimes occur immediately after birth as a result of weakness in the respiratory musculature, the tongue, and the mastication and swallowing muscles; including cyanosis, aspiration and respiratory-tract infections, and difficulties with feeding.

Muscle biopsy shows that type-1 fibres predominate in 75 per cent of cases. Groups of small rod- and thread-shaped structures (rods) are present — often in the subsarcolemmal region — in both type-1 and type-2 fibres. The name nemaline myopathy was chosen on account of the Greek word for thread (nema). Other authors prefer the name 'rod disease'.

Electron microscopy has shown that the rods derive from the Z-discs. Some biopsies may show rods in all fibres while other biopsies may contain a few fibres with rods. It has been shown that no correlation exists between the number of fibres with rods and the severity of the illness. Furthermore, rods do not appear to be specific for nemaline myopathy: they can be observed in numerous neuromuscular diseases, including other congenital myopathies (such as central core disease, multicore disease and congenital fibre-type disproportion). The clinically normal heterozygotes in the recessive form of the disease can usually be identified because they also have rods in the muscle fibres.

Centronuclear and myotubular myopathies

These congenital myopathies form a group which includes the autosomal recessive and autosomal dominant as well as the sporadic forms. The facial and extraocular muscles are affected in about half the patients. Fibres with a centrally located nucleus in which the normally present subsarcolemmal nuclei are frequently absent can be seen in transverse sections of the muscle biopsy. There is a marked variation in the number of fibres with central nuclei, not only between patients but also between biopsies from different muscles in the same patient. Sometimes the centrally located myofibrils are absent and then the fibres resemble myotubules when examined by light microscopy; hence the name myotubular myopathy. Sometimes type-1 fibres with a small diameter are observed as well. Such findings gave rise to other names, for example, type-1 fibre atrophy with central nuclei.

The X-linked myotubular myopathy (also called type-1-fibre hypotrophy with central nuclei by other authors) forms a clear clinical entity. There is a marked variation in expressivity of the clinical picture; sometimes it is so severe that the patient dies as early as one or two days after birth. Reduced fetal movements and hydramnion occur frequently during the pregnancy. The infants are cyanotic immediately after birth because of respiratory insufficiency. If they survive this stage they show a non-progressive, generalized muscle weakness, which may involve the facial and extraocular muscles. Muscle fibres resembling myotubules and small (hypotrophic) type-1 fibres are not only found in these patients but may also be found scattered between the normal fibres in the carriers.

Congenital fibre-type disproportion

Children with this condition have hypotonia and generalized muscle weakness immediately after birth. Contractures and multiple deformations of the skeleton such as hip dislocation, kyphoscoliosis and varus and valgus deformities of the feet are common. Although there is an initial increase in muscle weakness, after several years the condition stabilizes. Sometimes the weakness can even be seen to improve. The children are often abnormally small for their age. The muscle biopsy shows that the type-1 fibres are smaller than the type-2 fibres (disproportion of fibre type sizes). Half the cases show more type-1 than type-2 fibres (type-1-fibre predominance). This condition is more likely to be a syndrome than a disease.

Multicore disease

This condition shows numerous small areas (5–10 μm in diameter) with loss of cross-striations. Electron microscopy has shown that there is not only a disintegration of the sarcomeres with streaming of the Z-lines but also a reduction or absence of mitochondria in these areas.

If there are many areas with a very small diameter (1–3 μm) one speaks of minicore disease. This condition appears to be extremely rare. If the lesions are much bigger (35–75 μm) and if they also contain vesicular nuclei then one speaks of a focal loss of cross-striations. Extraocular muscles are often involved in this condition and the clinical picture is frequently progressive. Sometimes all three lesions may show up in the same muscle biopsy or the same muscle fibre, in which case it is difficult to establish a definite diagnosis on the basis of histopathology.

Sometimes the signs of multicore disease are not present immediately after birth, developing later in childhood or in adult life. It is quite likely that multicore disease does not represent a disease entity. The existence of different modes of inheritance strengthens this argument; both autosomal recessive and dominant forms of the condition have been described.

Postscript

The names of congenital myopathies date from the time when muscle biopsies were considered essential for a diagnosis.

Many patients with congential myopathy have hip dislocation. It would be good practice, therefore, in every baby with congenital dislocation of the hip, to think of a congenital myopathy as the cause of dislocation.

X-linked myotubular myopathy is often a serious disease. Carriers of this disease can often be identified.

Parents of children with congenital myopathy automatically think of a wheelchair. The physician in charge must not make this mistake.

18
Myopathies with abnormal mitochondria

The first description of a patient suffering from a myopathy in which abnormal mitochondria were present in the muscle fibres was given by Luft *et al.* (1962). This patient also had signs of serious hypermetabolism which did not appear to be due to hyperthyroidism. Since that time a large number of patients with muscle weakness and morphologically abnormal mitochondria have been described. These diseases are also known as 'mitochondrial myopathies'.

Electron microscopy of the muscle fibres — especially those in the subsarcolemmal region — reveals the presence of too many mitochondria. These mitochondria are abnormal in shape and size and often contain paracrystalline inclusions. If muscle sections are stained by the modified Gomori-trichrome method and examined by light microscopy, the subsarcolemmal areas are coloured bright red. This gives the fibres an irregular ragged aspect in transverse section, thus they are known as 'ragged red fibres'. The number of ragged red fibres in the section varies, but not all fibres are affected at the same time. These ragged red fibres are less specific for mitochondrial myopathies than was originally thought. Sometimes they are seen in neuromuscular diseases which are not considered to belong to mitochondrial myopathies (for example, myotonic dystrophy, polymyositis, acid maltase deficiency, etc.).

The classification of mitochondrial myopathies on morphological grounds proved unsatisfactory. On the one hand the mitochondria were not only morphologically abnormal but also functionally abnormal. On the other hand, morphologically normal muscle mitochondria were found in which the mitochondrial metabolism was abnormal (e.g. carnitine palmityltransferase deficiency). Thus the group of mitochondrial myopathies, although originally discovered by the morphologists, gradually became the indisputable territory of biochemists (Table 18.1). In this context it became apparent that the mitochondrial defect was not restricted to muscle tissue; several other organs could be involved, or it could be systemic.

Clinically speaking, the mitochondrial myopathies form a particularly heterogenous group. They can occur at any age, from

Table 18.1 Biochemical classification of mitochondrial defects. According to Scholte (1986).

1.	*Oxidative phosphorylation defects.*
(a)	*Respiratory chain (electron transport) defects.*
	NADH-CoQ reductase deficiency.
	Ubiquinone deficiency.
	Cytochrome bc_1 deficiency.
	Cytochrome aa_3 deficiency.
(b)	*Phosphorylation defects.*
	ATP-synthetase deficiency (Mg^{2+}-ATPase deficiency).
	Adenine nucleotide translocator inhibition.[1]
	Proton-pumping defect at site 1, 2, or 3.
	Loose coupling.[1]
2.	*Dehydrogenase defects.*
(a)	*Acyl-CoA dehydrogenase deficiencies.*
	Acyl-CoA dehydrogenase deficiency due to deficiency of electron transport flavoprotein (ETF).
	Multiple acyl-CoA dehydrogenase deficiency due to ETF-dehydrogenase deficiency.
	Long-chain fatty acyl-CoA dehydrogenase deficiency.
	Medium-chain fatty acyl-CoA dehydrogenase deficiency.
	Butyryl-CoA dehydrogenase deficiency.
	Glutaryl-CoA dehydrogenase deficiency.
	Isovaleryl-CoA dehydrogenase deficiency.
(b)	*Deficiencies of dehydrogenases with acyl-CoA as product.*
	Pyruvate dehydrogenase deficiency.
	Pyruvate dehydrogenase phosphatase deficiency.

Dihydrolipoyl transacetylase deficiency.
2-Ketoglutarate dehydrogenase deficiency.
Branched-chain ketoacid dehydrogenase deficiency.
Lipoamide dehydrogenase deficiency.

(c) *Deficiencies of dehydrogenases not related to CoA metabolism.*
Glutamate dehydrogenase deficiency.
Glycine cleavage enzyme deficiency.
Sarcosine dehydrogenase deficiency.

3. *Transport defects.*
(a) *Defects in the carnitine system for acyl-transport.*
Carnitine deficiency.[1]
Carnitine palmityl transferase I deficiency.
Acylcarnitine–carnitine translocase deficiency.
Carnitine palmityltransferase II deficiency.
Combined CPT I and II deficiency.
Carnitine acetyltransferase deficiency.

(b) *Transport defects not related to the carnitine system.*
Pyruvate translocator defect.
Ornithine translocator defect.

4. *Defective synthesis of oxidative substrates* (non-redox reactions).
Multiple carboxylase deficiency due to biotinidase deficiency.
Multiple carboxylase deficiency due to holocarboxylase synthetase deficiency.
Propionyl-CoA carboxylase deficiency.
Pyruvate carboxylase deficiency.
3-Methyl-crotonoyl-CoA carboxylase deficiency.
Methyl-malonyl-CoA mutase deficiency.
3-Keto-acyl-CoA transferase deficiency.
Acetoacetyl-CoA thiolase deficiency.
2-Methyl-acetoacetyl-CoA thiolase deficiency.
Malonyl-CoA decarboxylase deficiency.

5. *Defect in general mitochondrial biosynthesis.*

6. *Defects not directly linked to mitochondrial ATP production.*
Carbamoyl phosphate synthetase deficiency.
N-Acetylglutamate synthetase deficiency.
Ornithine transcarbamoylase deficiency.
Ferrochelatase deficiency.

---

[1] Probably secondary to another mitochondrial defect.

birth to the sixties. Although various modes of inheritance have been described, in most patients no heredity has been established (sporadic cases).

The muscle weakness may be generalized or manifest itself as a limb-girdle syndrome, a facioscapulohumeral syndrome, progressive external ophthalmoplegia, or a distal condition. It is remarkable that many patients become fatigued after relatively light muscular exercise. This exercise intolerance can sometimes precede complaints about muscle weakness by months or even years. Many patients also have an increased lactate concentration in the blood. Most mitochondrial myopathies have only been described in one or a few patients, each of whom has shown markedly different (clinical) aspects. Clinically, therefore, it is impossible to diagnose mitochondrial myopathy; at best it can be suspected and, in the end, only the morphological and biochemical examination of the muscle biopsy may confirm the diagnosis. Often there are more systems involved and all kinds of other signs may occur, for example, delayed growth, congenital cataract, hypoglycaemia, etc. Oculocraniosomatic neuromuscular disease (Kearns–Sayre syndrome, see p. 91) is an example of such a multisystem condition. The central nervous system is often also involved in the pathological process; in this case signs of cerebral involvement may predominate over those of muscular involvement ('mitochondrial encephalomyopathies').

Postscript

It is impossible to give a clinical diagnosis of mitochondrial myopathy because it can begin at any age, because it can be hereditary or non-hereditary, and because the weakness can manifest itself in any muscle of the body. For the same reasons it should, however, always be kept in mind.

An increased serum lactate concentration in a patient with muscle weakness may indicate a mitochondrial myopathy.

Not every patient with a mitochondrial myopathy has an increased serum lactate concentration.

Every patient with mitochondrial myopathy differs from another.

19

Myotonic disorders

The myotonic disorders consist of a group of non-related hereditary neuromuscular diseases. Each has the presence of myotonia in common (Table 19.1), but one may distinguish between action myotonia, percussion myotonia, and electromyographic myotonia.

Action and percussion myotonia manifest themselves in the form of delayed relaxation after muscle contraction. Action myotonia can be observed after a patient has strongly tightened a muscle. Percussion myotonia develops after a muscle contraction has been elicited by mechanical stimulation, in this case a short, hard blow with the percussion hammer on the muscle involved. Percussion myotonia is often missed by the inexperienced clinician because the blow with the percussion hammer was not hard enough. In most cases action myotonia can be elicited by asking the patient to clench his fist tightly and then to release it quickly: as a result of the delay in contraction it will take quite a bit of time before the thumb and the fingers are fully extended again. If this process is repeated several times by the patient there is a clear tendency for the myotonia to decrease or disappear. Sometimes, however, the opposite happens and the myotonia is seen to

Table 19.1. Diseases associated with myotonia.

Myotonic dystrophy (Steinert's disease); autosomal dominant.
Myotonia congenita:
— autosomal dominant *(Thomsen's disease).*
— autosomal recessive *(Becker).*
Familial periodic paralysis; autosomal dominant:
— hyperkalaemic form, also called paramyotonia congenita (Eulenburg) or adynamia episodica hereditaria (Gamstorp).
— hypokalaemic form.
Chondrodystrophic myotonia (Schwartz–Jampel syndrome); autosomal recessive; onset in first years of life and associated with skeletal deformities, joint contractures, facial and ocular abnormalities, a high-pitched voice and a generalized hypertrophy of the muscles.

increase; this phenomenon (myotonia paradoxa) occurs mostly in paramyotonia congenita.

Percussion myotonia can be elicited best by percussion of the thenar eminence with a percussion hammer; this immediately results in a long-lasting flexion and opposition of the thumb — complete relaxation takes many seconds. In fact it is possible to elicit percussion myotonia in every muscle, although the effect is usually less marked than in the thenar eminence: often it only produces a local muscle contraction. Although percussion myotonia can also be elicited in the tongue, this muscle is not very suitable. The patient often experiences the hard blow as unpleasant because the protruding tongue rests on the teeth; he will be inclined to withdraw his tongue thus making it hard for the examiner to observe the local contraction. If, nevertheless, one still wants to elicit this phenomenon it is best to place a spatula between the tongue and the lower teeth.

Electromyography in myotonic disorders reveals high-frequency repetitive discharges which first increase in frequency and amplitude and then rapidly diminish. This activity can be heard through a loudspeaker. First there is a very characteristic increase in volume and then a rapid reduction (dive-bomber effect).

Electromyographic myotonia can be evoked by moving the needle-electrode, or it can be observed after percussion or contraction of the muscle. One must bear in mind that electromyographic myotonia can also occur in diseases without action and/or percussion myotonia, for example in denervation, polymyositis or acid maltase deficiency. The exact pathophysiology of myotonia is unknown, although it is generally assumed that the origin of the phenomenon must be sought in the muscle itself, as is indicated by its persistence following curarization or after blockage of the peripheral nerve.

Myotonic dystrophy

Myotonic dystrophy, also named dystrophia myotonica or Steinert's disease, is probably one of the most frequent neuromuscular diseases in the West. The gene responsible for this autosomal dominant disease is located on chromosome 19.

It is generally assumed that the first symptoms and signs begin between the ages of 15 and 30. Often, it is difficult for the patient to indicate when exactly his first complaints or signs began. The onset of the disease is probably more frequent during adolescence than in later life. Some patients have minor complaints, for example, patients who only have a cataract and/or alopecia. There are also patients who show myotonia after making a fist but who hardly see anything unusual in this phenomenon; all the more so because they have 'had it for ages' and other members of the family have it as well. It is estimated that half the patients are unaware that they are suffering from the disease, in spite of clear clinical signs. General practitioners may have a patient with myotonic dystrophy without being aware of it, while a neurologist will have missed a case of myotonic dystrophy at least once in his life.

Myotonic dystrophy can be considered a multisystemic condition (Table 19.2). Myotonia can be observed in three different ways, viz. after contraction of the muscle (action myotonia), after percussion of the muscle by means of a percussion hammer (percussion myotonia) and by means of electromyography (see above). Action myotonia in myotonia dystrophy occurs when clenching the fist. If the patient is asked to open his hand rapidly it takes many seconds for the muscles to relax. Fully stretching the thumb appears to be especially difficult. Patients rarely complain about their action myotonia, which is never painful. Action myotonia shows a tendency to worsen in cold weather and to improve in a warm environment or after several contractions and relaxations.

Percussion myotonia can occur in the thenar eminence; it is often associated with adduction and opposition of the thumb. A local contraction after percussion can often be observed in the m.abductor digiti minimi and in the lower arm extensors, less often in the m.biceps brachii, the tongue, the m.quadriceps femoris, and the calves, and relatively rarely in other muscles. The muscle weakness and wasting are especially common in the face and distal musculature of the limbs. As soon as the patient enters the examination room, weakness of the facial muscles and ptosis can be seen (Fig. 19.1), as well as atrophy of the temporalis and the masseter muscles.

Examination may reveal that the weakness of the mm.orbicularis oculi is greater than the weakness of the other facial muscles. The sternocleidomastoid muscles are often very atrophic and weak as

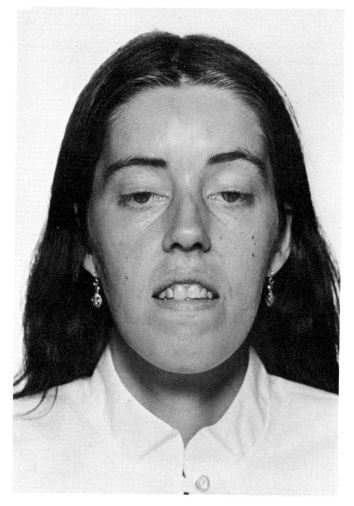

Fig. 19.1. Myotonic dystrophy. The facial appearance is characteristic. There is a lack of facial expression, ptosis, atrophy of the mm.temporales and an open-hanging mouth, due to sagging of the jaw.

well (Fig. 19.2). The hand and feet extensors and the small muscles of the hands are also affected (Fig. 19.3), but the muscles of the shoulder and pelvic girdle are rarely weakened. The myotonia becomes less marked with an increase in the weakness

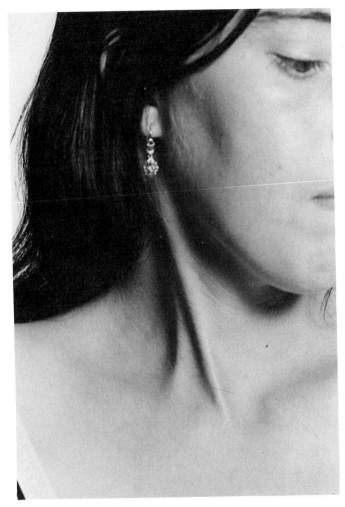

Fig. 19.2. Myotonic dystrophy. Marked atrophy of the m.sternocleido-mastoideus.

and atrophy of the lower arm and hand muscles. Many patients have a more or less pronounced nasal and dysarthric speech, not only because of facial weakness but also because the palate, tongue and pharynx are affected.

The myotatic reflexes are poor or absent, and sometimes this does not correlate with the seriousness of the weakness or atrophy.

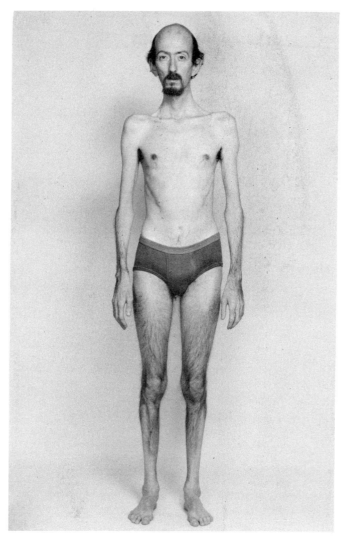

Fig. 19.3. Myotonic dystrophy. Inspection of the patient shows fronto-parietal balding, and atrophy of the temporal and masseter muscles and of the distal musculature of the limbs.

Table 19.2. Principal abnormalities in myotonic dystrophy.

Skeletal muscles.
Weakness and atrophy of the m.temporalis, m.masseter, facial muscles, m.levator palpebrae, palate, pharynx, m.sternocleidomastoideus, diaphragm and distal muscles of the limbs; myotonia after making a fist and after percussion of the thenar and hypothenar eminences, the extensor muscles of the forearms and the calves.

Heart muscle.
Arrhythmias (atrium, ventricle); conduction defects (prolonged PR interval, QRS widening.

Smooth muscles.
Oesophagus (dysphagia); colon (abdominal pain, diarrhoea, constipation, rarely megacolon); gallbladder (gallstones); ciliary body (low intraocular tension).

Eye.
Lens (characteristic cataract); retina (peripheral pigmentary changes, abnormal electroretinogram).

Hair.
Frontoparietal balding, especially in men; less frequent and less marked in women.

Endocrine glands.
Testicular atrophy; pancreas (hypersecretion of insulin after glucose administration, abnormalities in glucose tolerance test, rarely clinical diabetes); thyroid (very rarely hypo- or hyperthyroidism).

Brain.
Low IQ; mental retardation in neonatal form; hypersomnia; lack of drive.

Peripheral nerves.
Rarely, low motor conduction velocities of the n.peroneus or clinical signs of polyneuropathy.

Skeletal.
Hyperostosis frontalis interna; diffuse hyperostosis; large frontal sinuses; small sella turcica; ossification of the diaphragma sella.

Lungs.
Alveolar hyperventilation.

Frontoparietal balding is found more or less regularly, especially in men (see Fig. 19.3). Testicular atrophy, accompanied by a reduced spermatogenesis, is also seen in 60–80 per cent of male patients.

Women, on the other hand, rarely show gonadal disorders although the rate of abortion and neonatal death occurs two to three times more often than in a control group.

A strong, rapid, and persistent increase in insulin after the oral administration of glucose occurs in an estimated 60 per cent of patients. Abnormal glucose tolerance tests with flattened or diabetic curves, as well as clinical diabetes, are observed less often.

A very typical cataract can be observed by means of a slit-lamp; white or coloured opacities are mainly subcapsular with the central part of the lens remaining relatively unaffected. The incidence of this cataract increases with age, in patients over 50 it is almost 100 per cent.

It is estimated that mental retardation occurs in 40 per cent of the patients. A combination of distal muscle weakness (hands) and mental retardation may mean a further social slide for the patient and his family. Many patients show lack of drive and initiative, and hypersomnia; this sometimes resembles narcolepsy, with patients falling asleep in the daytime.

As a rule, clinical signs of cardiac involvement are not prominent, although electrocardiographic abnormalities are found in about 80 per cent of patients. These consist of arrhythmias and disturbances of atrioventricular conduction, in particular a prolonged PR interval (> 0.20 seconds) and a widened QRS complex (> 0.08 seconds).

Respiratory difficulties may occur, not only as a result of weakness and myotonia of the respiratory musculature (including the diaphragm) and swallowing difficulties with aspiration, but also because of alveolar hypoventilation. Patients with myotonic dystrophy are a high-risk group with regard to anaesthesia, because of unsuspected cardiac conduction disorders and arrhythmias, as well as lung function impairment. Some patients appear to be hypersensitive to thiopentone and develop respiratory depression and apnoea.

Radiological changes in the skull are observed frequently, including hyperostosis frontalis interna, which may be combined with a more diffuse hyperostosis of the calvarium, a small sella turcica, sometimes with calcification of the diaphragma sellae, and large frontal sinuses.

Electromyography usually contributes little to the diagnosis. Electromyographic myotonia is rarely found without clinical signs of myotonia (in retrospect the neurological examination usually appears to have been insufficient on this point). Neither short-duration, low-voltage action potentials nor electromyographic myotonia are characteristic of myotonic dystrophy.

Serum creatine kinase activity is usually normal or slightly increased and for that reason does not provide any help with the diagnosis. The muscle biopsy shows variation in fibre diameter, an increase in fibres with internal nuclei — often accompanied by the formation of nuclear chains — and often ringed fibres and sarcoplasmic masses. Sometimes one can observe single or small groups of angular small-diameter fibres with high oxidative enzyme activity and non-specific esterase activity, which tally in all respects with the abnormalities observed in denervation. Because of these neurogenic findings, some authors prefer the name myotonic atrophy. In muscles which are only slightly affected one can sometimes observe type-1 fibre atrophy.

Finally, some muscle spindles may show numerous very small intrafusal muscle fibres due to longitudinal splitting. In spite of these many histopathological changes, it is hardly ever necessary, in practice, to carry out a muscle biopsy. At most the findings can confirm the diagnosis already established by clinical examination.

Frequently a member of a family who requests genetic counselling wishes to know whether he/she is also suffering from the disease. The identification of heterozygotes before the age of 20 is much more difficult than it is later, because an older patient will probably already have manifest signs of the disease. Heterozygotes can be identified by careful neurological examination and a slit-lamp examination carried out by an experienced ophthalmologist. No other examination methods (determination of serum creatine kinase activity, electromyography, muscle biopsy, etc.) provide better information. In some cases a linkage investigation may help identification, both prenatal (amniocentesis) and postnatal (saliva investigation). This technique is based on knowledge of the fact that both the gene for myotonic dystrophy and the secretor gene are located close together on the same chromosome. To have any predictive value, however, both the parents as well as several generations of the family must be available for examination. If the patient is found to be suffering from the disease then each child runs a 50 per cent risk of contracting the disease too. It is sometimes pointed out that the disease occurs at a younger age and is more serious in each subsequent generation. This is very unlikely and, if it does occur, it is very exceptional. The presence of a congenital form in mothers only slightly affected with the disease themselves may partially explain this phenomenon.

Congenital myotonic dystrophy

This is a separate clinical entity which is also called neonatal, infantile or early onset myotonic dystrophy, and myotonic dysembryoplasia. A phenomenon not fully understood is that the congenital form only occurs in children of mothers with myotonic dystrophy. Consequently, examination of the mother, who usually shows only minor signs of the disease, represents the final chapter in this diagnosis.

The most careful investigations regarding congenital myotonic dystrophy were carried out by Harper. About half the mothers he examined felt little fetal movement during pregnancy and about half also had hydramnios during the last months of pregnancy. Hydramnios is caused by failure of the fetus to swallow. Both signs, hydramnios and reduced fetal movement, may also, for that matter, occur in other congenital myopathies.

Immediately after birth the children show a serious generalized hypotonia and bilateral facial weakness which leads to difficulties with sucking. The shortened median part of the upper lip gives it the appearance of an inverted V. This characteristic tented upper lip has also been compared to the mouth of a carp or shark. Serious respiratory difficulties can occur in the first hours to days after birth, which is why many babies die during this period. Respiratory difficulties are based on involvement of the intercostal muscles and diaphragm; the latter can also be shown by X-ray (raised diaphragm, especially on the right-hand side). Apart from this, pulmonary immaturity and aspiration pneumonia also play a role. If these phenomena are recognized in an early phase and treated adequately then few further lung complications are observed after the first month. If the children survive the first few weeks after birth many other signs may follow. Half the patients have talipes, but a minority show other deformations and contractures as well; presenting the syndrome of arthrogryposis multiplex congenita. Motor development is also delayed, partly because of the existing foot deformations. The children will, however, always learn to walk. Mental retardation is seen in about 70 per cent of children. Nasal and dysarthric speech is usually present. Strabismus is also observed relatively frequently.

The serious hypotonia will gradually disappear and distal muscular weakness becomes manifest. It is important to bear in mind that clinical myotonia does not occur in the first 12 months, rarely occurs below the age of 5 but is almost always present after 10 years of age. If the infant shows mainly clinical myotonia then the diagnosis of congenital myotonic dystrophy may be rejected: in this case the patient very likely suffers from the autosomal dominant form of myotonia congenita (Thomsen's disease). There are some observations of electromyographic myotonia in neonates with congenital myotonic dystrophy but, in general, EMG is not found to contribute much to the diagnosis.

The therapy of myotonic dystrophy, often a relatively benign disease with slow progression, remains palliative. Respiratory exercises are indicated for patients who show signs of alveolar hypoventilation and other respiratory difficulties. Generally, patients do not tend to develop contractures. Many patients experience difficulty with walking as a result of dropfoot. This difficulty can be alleviated to a large extent by firm ankle-high boots or ankle–foot arthrodesis. As patients rarely complain about myotonia there is, as a rule, no need for drugs. Since cardiac abnormalities, especially conduction defects, are often present, quinine and procainamide are in fact contraindicated. On the other hand it is safe to give phenytoin orally, in a dose of 100 mg 3–4 times daily.

Myotonia congenita

Although the autosomal dominant type of myotonia congenita (or Thomsen's disease) was described first and for that reason is perhaps best known, the autosomal recessive type — described by Becker — is also often observed. Myotonia and muscle hypertrophy are the main signs in both types. In autosomal dominant myotonia congenita the first signs occur as early as in infancy. Sometimes the mother will notice that her baby has the disease: the child's eyes when closed tightly as a result of coughing or sneezing will take longer to open again due to myotonia of the mm.orbiculares oculi. Action and percussion myotonia (see p. 107) may occur in almost any muscle. These signs tend to increase during puberty and in later life their intensity will usually decrease again. The myotonia, however, can also vary from day to day or within the same day; it is often adversely affected by prolonged resting, menstruation, pregnancy, fatigue, stress, and possibly also by cold surroundings. Improvement can be obtained by repeated muscle contractions. Myotonia can be provoked by asking the patient to close his eyes tightly or to clench his fist, it can also be elicited by asking him to look up for a long time (which causes contraction of the m.levator palpebrae) and then to lower his eyes again. This will give rise to a slow relaxation of the upper eye lids (myotonic lid lag).

Patients can be seriously handicapped in their daily activities as a result of limb myotonia. Patients may develop myotonia in all muscles and then fall over as stiff as a plank as a result of sudden movement (e.g. stumbling) or when given a fright. It is obvious that this phenomenon of literally freezing with fright can be fatal if driving a car. Although the myotonia is usually painless the occurrence of pain has been described in some families.

Hypertrophy may be observed in the neck muscles as well as in the m.deltoideus, the m.biceps brachii, the m.triceps brachii, the m.quadriceps femoris and the m.gastrocnemius. A generalized hypertrophy can also be observed; this makes the patient look athletic, although usually without the muscle power suggested by such an appearance. Myotatic reflexes are normal. Serum creatine kinase activity is also normal and the muscle biopsy shows no or only aspecific changes.

Autosomal recessive myotonia congenita

This manifests itself in childhood or later, particularly in the muscles of the legs. Gradually the symptoms will spread to the other muscles so that, by the time the child has grown up, a generalized myotonia is usually present. It is often worse than in Thomsen's disease. The fact that minor muscle weakness and wasting may also develop is important, especially when considering the differential diagnosis with myotonic dystrophy.

The treatment for both types of myotonia congenita consists of 100 mg phenytoin 3–4 times daily or 1 g procainamide 3–4 times daily. If this does not show any effect, 250 mg acetazolamide 2–3 times daily or a combination of the above medications can be tried. In addition, a daily dose of 20 mg N-propyl-Ajmalin or taurine (100–150 mg per kg body weight) are also recommended. Even then results are often disappointing and the favourable effect may only last a short time.

Postscript

Myotonic dystrophy occurs much more frequently than one thinks.

The diagnosis of myotonic dystrophy is missed more often than one thinks.

Many patients say that the disease does not occur in their family. Don't believe it.

The best way of diagnosing myotonic dystrophy is by a neurological and slit-lamp examination. All other investigations, including EMG and muscle biopsy, can only confirm a clinically established diagnosis and, therefore, are superfluous.

A cataract is pathognomonic for dystrophia myotonica. One must look closely into the patient's eyes (with a slit-lamp).

After percussion of the thenar eminence in healthy people, irregular contractions causing movement may be observed. In genuine myotonia, however, the contracted thenar muscles relax very slowly.

Many patients with myotonic dystrophy are better off with money than with medicine.

20

Glycogen storage diseases

In many glycogen storage diseases there is a dysfunction of the energy supply to the skeletal muscles. The principal signs in some of these diseases are muscular pain, cramp, and stiffness after exercise. The clinical picture is sometimes characterized by muscle weakness. The signs and symptoms are caused by enzyme deficiencies which inhibit glycogen metabolism. In an early numerical classification by Cori, acid maltase deficiency, for example, used to be mentioned: 'type II-glycogenose'. This meaningless, sometimes confusing and error-inducing nomenclature has now been replaced by a classification based on the underlying enzyme deficiency (Table 20.1).

Acid maltase deficiency

This autosomal recessive condition may present several months after birth (infantile type or Pompe's disease) or may become manifest in later life (adult type). The gene for the disease is located at the long arm of chromosome 17.

A patient with Pompe's disease stores glycogen in the skeletal muscles, but also in many other organs, for instance, the heart, the liver, and the central and peripheral nervous systems. The children are markedly hypotonic, and besides generalized muscle weakness also show enlargement of the tongue, heart and liver. The disease is gradually progressive and the patients usually die of cardiac or respiratory complications in the first year of life.

The adult type of acid maltase deficiency is possibly the most frequently occurring type of glycogen storage disease associated with myopathy. A carefully recorded history will often show that as children most patients had the kind of difficulties associated with neuromuscular disease: poor performance during gymnastics classes, never being able to run as fast as most of the other children in the class, no interest in sport, and so on. Weakness which affects the proximal muscle groups more than the distal muscles, and the

Table 20.1 The glycogenoses.

Type	Enzyme deficiency	Synonym
I	Glucose-6-phosphatase.*	Von Gierke's disease
II	Acid maltase (acid alpha-1,4-glucosidase).	Pompe's disease.
III	Debranching enzyme** (amylo-1,6-glucosidase).	Cori's disease. Forbes' disease. Limit dextrinosis.
IV	Branching enzyme (amylo-1,4→1,6-transglucosidase; alpha-1,4-glucan 6-glycosyltransferase).	Andersen's disease Amylopectinosis.
V	Muscle phosphorylase.**	McArdle's disease.
VI	Liver phosphorylase.*	Hers' disease.
VII	Phosphofructokinase.**	Tarui's disease.
VIII	Liver phosphorylase-b-kinase: Phosphoglycerate-kinase.** Phosphoglycerate-mutase.** Lactate-dehydrogenase-M-subunit.**	

* The muscles are hardly ever affected in these diseases.
** In these diseases there is no increase in lactic acid in the venous blood after ischaemic muscle exercise.

muscles of the pelvic girdle more than those of the shoulder girdle will gradually develop in early adulthood.

Besides a limb-girdle syndrome, respiratory failure may also occur. Several patients have been described who were first admitted to a general ward with severe respiratory distress, which later appeared to be due to an acid maltase deficiency with involvement of the diaphragm and other respiratory muscles.

As so often in medicine, the diagnosis is easy once it is thought of (Table 20.2). Serum creatine kinase activity is usually slightly raised. The electromyogram shows abnormal irritability of the muscles with high-frequency and myotonic discharges as well as fibrillation potentials and short positive waves. Of practical importance is the fact that these bizarre high-frequency discharges are sometimes found exclusively in the paraspinal muscles.

Although myotonic discharges may be seen in the EMG, clinical signs of myotonia are never observed.

In the biopsy, small vacuoles, often filled with glycogen as well as showing high acid phosphatase activity (a lysosomal enzyme), are often observed in several or many of the muscle fibres. Biochemical identification of acid maltase deficiency in muscle tissue confirms the diagnosis. The deficiency can also be demonstrated in the leucocytes. Finally, it appears that the excretion of acid maltase in urine has decreased. The disease progresses slowly and it is therefore relatively benign. Most patients, however, are seriously handicapped and require the use of a wheelchair by the time they are 60 years of age.

Heterozygotes can often be identified by determining the acid maltase activity in muscle tissue, cultured fibroblasts, leucocytes, or urine. This may be important in the genetic counselling of healthy relatives of patients with this disease.

No drugs are able to treat the consequences of enzyme defici-

Table 20.2 Diagnosing acid maltase deficiency in a patient with a limb-girdle syndrome.

(1) Think of this diagnosis as one of the alternatives	
(2) Leucocytes	– decreased activity of acid maltase.
(3) Urine	– decreased excretion of acid maltase.
(4) Muscle tissue	– histopathology: vacuoles with high acid phosphatase activity and accumulation of glycogen.
	– biochemistry: acid maltase deficiency.
	– tissue culture shows identical morphological and biochemical abnormalities.
(5) EMG	– pay particular attention to the paraspinal muscles: bizarre repetitive discharges, positive waves, myotonic discharges.
(6) Serum creatine kinase activity mildly raised	

ency on glycogen metabolism. On the other hand, patients can often be helped considerably with postural exercises, especially since disease progression is slow. In addition, the treatment of pes equinus is also important.

Muscle phosphorylase deficiency

This condition is also called McArdle's disease. As a result of myophosphorylase deficiency, glycogen cannot be broken down and is thus unavailable as a source of energy in case of strenuous physical exercise.

The first signs of this disease are often observed in childhood; the patient will tire easily with heavy physical exercise. Gradually, the patient develops a muscular ache in the legs which increases over the years. Finally, severe and painful muscle cramps will occur after relatively minor muscular exercise. These cramps may persist for hours. Occasionally, there are episodes in which the urine is dark brown (myoglobinuria, see also p. 144) several hours after severe exercise. This sign is rarely noticed after the age of 40. Cramp and stiffness may occur in any muscle which is used intensively, although it usually occurs in the muscles of the lower limbs. In classic cases, the patient will say that he is able to walk unassisted for quite some time provided the ground is level. As soon as he has to walk up an incline he becomes fatigued and develops painful cramps in his legs. If the patient slows down, walking becomes easier and can be kept up for a longer period of time (second-wind phenomenon). It is not easy to explain this phenomenon. Some authors have suggested that the free fatty acids in the blood are used as a source of energy for muscular exercise while others believe an augmented or altered distribution of blood flow to the muscles to be responsible. Although the patients show no weakness or any other neurological abnormality between attacks, a permanent weakness of the proximal muscles may develop after middle-age (limb-girdle syndrome, see Table 14.1, p. 86). Serum creatine kinase is invariably raised, even at rest.

The diagnosis of McArdle's disease is usually indicated by observation of the way the muscles of the lower arm work under ischaemic conditions. Ischaemia can be achieved by increasing the pressure of a blood-pressure cuff around the upper arm to above arterial pressure, and then asking the patient to perform a certain amount of preferably standardized exercises with his lower arm and hand muscles. Healthy people can keep this up for several minutes, after which the power in the increasingly pale and numb lower arm gradually runs out. Eventually all muscle effort comes to a halt, although passive movement of the fingers and wrist remains possible. A patient with McArdle's disease will experience fatigue and disability after only a minute, with the fingers and wrist locked in a painful flexion contracture allowing neither passive nor active stretching. The contracture will persist for a long time after recovery of the circulation. Electromyography reveals no electrical activity in the maximal shortened muscle (true contracture). In healthy people, an increase in lactic acid in the venous blood of the lower arm can be seen about 3 minutes after the test. The lactate concentration before the test varies from 0.5–2.0 mmol/l; afterwards there is at least a threefold increase. As there is no glycogen breakdown in a patient with McArdle's disease during ischaemic muscle testing, there is no concomitant increase in lactic acid concentration either. In spite of being a good test for diagnostic purposes, ischaemic muscle testing is certainly not without risk for the patient (renal insufficiency as a result of myoglobinuria). Furthermore, the absence of an increase in lactic acid after ischaemic muscle testing is not specific for myophosphorylase deficiency, as it also occurs in several other glycogenoses (see Table 20.1). With this in mind, histochemical and biochemical analyses of a needle biopsy from the muscles of patients in whom this disease is suspected seems a better way of arriving at an accurate diagnosis.

Muscle biopsy will reveal subsarcolemmal accumulations of glycogen and a total lack of muscle phosphorylase activity in the muscle fibres. A biochemical examination confirming the phosphorylase deficiency in muscle tissue will confirm the diagnosis. There are actually two different types of this disease: one type with biochemically and immunologically absent myophosphorylase, and the other type with an enyzmatically inactive myophosphorylase protein that can be detected immunologically. Both types are autosomal recessive; an autosomal dominant form has also been described but this is extremely rare. The gene for myophosphorylase deficiency is located at the long arm of chromosome 11.

Some authors have found marked improvement of the complaint in patients given a long-term high-protein diet. No drug therapy is available. Although the disease usually has a relatively benign course — especially with a suitably adapted life-style — patients with acute renal insufficiency as a result of myoglobinuria have also been described.

Debranching-enzyme deficiency

Involvement of the muscles is rare in this autosomal recessive disease. In childhood the disease can manifest with hepatomegaly, hypoglycaemia, ketonuria, and growth retardation. The patients sometimes show generalized hypotonia and muscle weakness. They can recover completely from these after puberty, although the enzyme deficiency continues. Signs of the disease can recur at a later age with fatigue and cramps following muscle exercise. Proximal or distal muscle weakness have also been described.

A clear improvement was observed in a child treated with a high-protein and high-carbohydrate diet.

Branching-enzyme deficiency

In this very rare autosomal recessive disease there is an accumulation of abnormal glycogen resembling amylopectin. This abnormal polysaccharide is found, for example, in the cardiac muscle, the skeletal muscle (weakness, hypotonia, atrophy), the liver (hepatomegaly), the spleen (splenomegaly), and the lymph glands. The patients that have been described to date died before they were 4 years old.

Phosphofructokinase deficiency

This autosomal recessive condition must be considered very rare. The gene of phosphofructokinase deficiency is located at the long arm of chromosome 1. The signs and symptoms resemble those of McArdle's disease. In phosphofructokinase deficiency there is a blockage in the second stage of glycolysis. In recent years other conditions associated with a blockage at this stage have been described, as in phosphoglycerate kinase deficiency, phosphoglycerate mutase deficiency, and a deficiency of the M-subunit of lactate dehydrogenase. In all these conditions the patient complains of tiring easily and of experiencing cramps after strenuous muscle exercise. Myoglobinuria may also occur. No rise of venous lactate is seen after ischaemic forearm exercise.

21
Disorders of muscle lipid metabolism

In disorders of muscle lipid metabolism, storage of lipid in the muscle fibres often occurs. This may be caused by carnitine deficiency, but sometimes there is no known cause. A lipid-storage myopathy in patients with congenital ichthyosis, HBsAg-positive hepatitis, and mitochondrial abnormalities (mitochondria–lipid– glycogen (MLG) disease) has also been described.

Carnitine deficiency

Only a small amount of carnitine (gamma-trimethylamino-beta-hydroxybutyrate) is ingested (it is mainly found in fish and meat); most of it is synthesized in the liver from lysine. From the liver the carnitine is delivered, via the blood, to the different organs, including the muscles. A carnitine deficiency of the muscle can therefore be the result of a defect in hepatic carnitine synthesis (systemic carnitine deficiency) or a defect in active carnitine transport from the extracellular fluid into the muscle (myopathic form of carnitine deficiency). It is actually quite possible that systemic carnitine deficiency is the result of a generalized defect in carnitine transport. As carnitine plays an important role in the transport of long-chain fatty acids to the mitochondria (where the fatty acids undergo beta-oxidation) carnitine deficiency will give rise to lipid storage. Physiologically, low serum carnitine concentrations are seen in pregnant women. Low serum carnitine concentrations are also found in severe cirrhosis of the liver — in this condition carnitine is deficient in the liver, the muscles, and in other organs. Low muscle carnitine concentrations occur in many neuromuscular diseases, but their values are never as low as in myopathic carnitine deficiency.

Systemic carnitine deficiency

This is probably an autosomal recessive disease. The first signs usually manifest themselves at a young age. They consist of one or more acute episodes of encephalopathy associated with liver insufficiency. The liver is enlarged and the attacks are preceded by nausea and vomiting, followed by stupor, confusion, and coma. During such attacks there is often metabolic acidosis. Muscle weakness may occur years before or after the signs of liver insufficiency. The proximal muscles are usually affected more than the distal musculature, although in principle, all muscles, including the muscles of the face, may be weak. As a rule, serum creatine kinase activity is slightly raised. The carnitine level is not only decreased in the serum but also in the liver, the muscle, and the heart. An accumulation of lipid is seen in the muscle fibres, especially the type-1 fibres.

Systemic carnitine deficiency has a poor prognosis, most patients dying before they are 20. Patients have also been described in whom the signs worsened in the last months of pregnancy or after giving birth. As therapy, DL-carnitine (2–8 g/day, administered orally) may be considered, although this only results in clinical improvement in some patients. Good results have also been reported with a daily oral administration of 10–100 mg riboflavin.

Myopathic carnitine deficiency

Usually sporadic, this condition may be autosomal recessive as well. The first signs can occur in early childhood or during adulthood. There is a progressive generalized muscle weakness and the proximal muscle groups are affected more than the distal musculature. The facial muscles are sometimes involved as well. Serum creatine kinase activity is usually slightly raised. Typically, the carnitine level is normal in serum, but lowered in muscle tissue. The muscle biopsy shows lipid accumulation, especially in type-I fibres.

The prognosis of myopathic carnitine deficiency is much better than that of the systemic form. Good results have been achieved with oral administration of DL-carnitine (2–8 g/day) and/or high doses of prednisone (100 mg/day). Propranolol (40 mg three times a day) gave good clinical improvement in several patients. Finally, some authors recommend that patients should be treated with a diet free of long-chain fatty acids.

Secondary carnitine deficiency syndromes

These can develop secondary to a variety of disorders, especially genetic defects of intermediary metabolism, often associated with organic aciduria. Secondary carnitine deficiency may manifest with muscle weakness, fatigue and episodes of vomiting. Improvements in these symptoms can sometimes be obtained by oral carnitine replacement therapy or administration of riboflavin.

Carnitine palmityltransferase deficiency

Carnitine palmityltransferase (CPT) is an enzyme which is located on both sides of the inner mitochondrial membrane. CPT I is on the outside of the inner membrane and catalyses the conversion of acyl-CoA into acylcarnitine. CPT II is located on the inside of the inner mitochondrial membrane and, in turn, converts the acyl-carnitine back into acyl-CoA, after which beta-oxidation takes place. Both CPT I and CPT II can be deficient and cause a clinical picture in which patients complain of attacks of severe muscle pain (myalgias) and a feeling of stiffness in the muscles (usually without real muscle cramps). This is often followed by myoglobinuria after several hours (see p. 144). At this stage muscle weakness may occur. The attacks are especially likely to occur after prolonged strenuous exercise and/or after fasting. Most of the patients are young men who, if questioned, appear to have been particularly prone to muscle pains in their teens.

Serum creatine kinase activity is increased during a period of muscle pain and myoglobinuria. The muscle biopsy, whether during or after an attack, is usually quite normal, although it may sometimes show a slight increase in lipids, especially in type-I fibres. Between attacks the patient does not show any abnormalities on neurological examination, serum creatine kinase activity is normal and, as a rule, the biopsy is also normal. The diagnosis can, therefore, only be established by carefully listening to the patient's history and by biochemical demonstration of a CPT deficiency in the muscle tissue.

The best therapy is a change in life-style. The patient must try not to do more than he is capable of or can tolerate. Furthermore, it is important to avoid long-term fasting. In the morning, particularly, he should not go too long without food. Frequent high-carbohydrate low-fat meals appear to aid patients.

Postscript

A patient with a carnitine deficiency myopathy stores lipid in the muscle fibres.

Not every patient with lipid storage in the muscle fibres has a carnitine deficiency myopathy.

A low serum carnitine concentration does not mean that the patient has a carnitine deficiency myopathy.

A patient may have a carnitine deficiency myopathy in spite of a normal serum carnitine concentration.

Not every patient with a myopathy and low muscle carnitine concentration has a carnitine deficiency myopathy.

So far, carnitine palmityltransferase deficiency is the only disorder of lipid metabolism in which the deficient enzyme is known. This disease, however, is not usually associated with muscle weakness or lipid storage in the muscle.

22

Periodic paralyses

Periodic paralyses are characterized by attacks of transient flaccid paralyses, especially of the muscles of the limbs. Recovery from the attacks is complete, but some patients may gradually develop permanent muscle weakness. This usually has the characteristics of a limb-girdle syndrome (see Table 14.1, p. 86). As well as autosomal dominant periodic paralyses, there are non-familial or sporadic forms (Table 22.1). A distinction is made between hypokalaemic and hyperkalaemic periodic paralyses.

Table 22.1. Periodic paralyses.

Autosomal dominant types.
  (1) Familial hypokalaemic periodic paralysis, most frequent type.
  (2) Familial hyperkalaemic periodic paralysis (synonyms: adynamia episodica hereditaria; paramyotonia congenita).
  (3) Familial normokalaemic periodic paralysis, very rare.
Non-hereditary, symptomatic (sporadic) types.
  (1) Hypokalaemic periodic paralysis.
    associated with thyrotoxicosis (especially in Asians).
    associated with thyroid hormone therapy.
    due to potassium loss as a result of:
    — hyperaldosteronism;
    — gastrointestinal disorders;
    — laxatives;
    — diuretics;
    — liquorice (glycyrrhizic acid);
    — carbenoxolone sodium.
  (2) Hyperkalaemic periodic paralysis.
    Addison's disease.
    Renal function disorders.
    Spironolactone.

A rare normokalaemic form has been described as well, although some authors doubt whether this disease exists. Although potassium is known to play a role, the actual pathogenesis of the condition remains unknown.

Efforts have been made to establish clinical differences between the hypo- and hyperkalaemic periodic paralyses. In this context it has been suggested that the hypokalaemic type occurs in puberty with attacks persisting for hours and occurring mostly at night or on waking in the morning, provoked by previous high-carbohydrate food intake or strenuous muscular exercise. The first hyperkalaemic attacks, on the other hand, occur as early as childhood; they are of short duration and usually occur in the daytime after a brief period of rest following muscular exercise. Nevertheless, many variations and deviations from these clinical patterns have been described; these are often associated with one particular family. Apart from this there appear to be such a sizeable overlap in signs between these conditions that it is often impossible to differentiate between them on clinical grounds.

Familial hypokalaemic periodic paralyses

This is the most frequently occurring type of periodic paralysis. Men are more often affected than women. The first attacks begin between 15 and 25 years of age. There is a marked variation in attack frequency: from several times a week to once a year. As a rule the number of attacks will increase until the age of 40 after which they will gradually decrease again; as a result many elderly patients no longer have any attacks. Attacks can be provoked by prolonged rest after strenuous muscular exercise, high-carbohydrate diet, alcohol, stress, and cold. The administration of corticosteroids, adrenalin, insulin, or glucose may also provoke an attack. The attacks usually occur at night or in the early hours of the morning when the patient wakes up with a symmetric flaccid paralysis of the muscles of the trunk and limbs. The bulbar and respiratory muscles are not usually affected. The patient perspires heavily and frequently, and complains of thirst (swallowing liquids remains possible). Minor attacks affect the proximal muscles of the legs in particular. During an attack the reflexes are diminished or absent. The duration of the attack varies from one hour to a week. Some patients are able to prevent or shorten the onset of an attack by keeping up light muscular activity, for example by continuously pacing up and down.

The diagnosis can be confirmed by determining the concentration of serum potassium during an attack. The low potassium level is also reflected in the electrocardiogram (flat T-waves, prominent U-waves, prolonged PR interval, widened QRS complex). Serum creatine kinase activity may be raised moderately or greatly during and immediately after the attack. As the attacks vary in frequency, intensity, and duration, in order to make a diagnosis, clinical observation of the patient while attempting to provoke an attack may be necessary. The best way to provoke an attack is to give the patient oral glucose (100 g) jointly with subcutaneous insulin (20 units). Next, check the potassium concentration every half-hour; it should decrease to at least 2.5 mEq/l. Electrocardiography should be performed throughout the test. An attack of muscle weakness associated with a decrease in potassium concentration confirms the diagnosis. However, the diagnosis should not be rejected out of hand if there is no attack. Sometimes a few hours pass before the insulin and glucose succeed in provoking an attack.

If a muscle biopsy is taken during or immediately after an attack, glycogen-filled vacuoles can be observed in the muscle fibres. These vacuoles disappear again after the attack. Before and after the attack, tubular aggregates can be seen in the type-II fibres: these are tube-like structures which develop as a result of proliferation of the sarcoplasmic reticulum. As a rule, no neurological abnormalities are observed between the attacks. Some authors, however, have noted myotonia in the upper eyelids (myotonic lid lag, see p. 118). After many attacks a permanent muscle weakness may develop in the legs and to a lesser extent in the arms.

An attack may be treated by the oral administration of 5–10 g potassium chloride which can be repeated after 1 hour if the desired effect is not achieved. To prevent attacks, 250 mg acetazolamide can be given 1–3 times a day. Even an improvement of permanent muscle weakness has been achieved with this treatment. The improvement is, however, often temporary, especially in older patients. In these patients one might try dichlorphenamide, a more potent carbonic anhydrase inhibitor, at a dosage of 50 mg, 2–3 times a day.

Familial hyperkalaemic periodic paralysis

This disease is also called adynamia episodica hereditaria, a name first used by the Swedish investigator Gamstorp. Many authors think that the paramyotonia congenita described by Eulenburg is identical with hyperkalaemic periodic paralysis and should be interpreted as a different expression of the same genetic defect. In this disease, attacks of myotonia and muscle weakness occur in cold conditions; the hands and face are particularly prone. In hyperkalaemic periodic paralysis the first attacks occur in childhood. The frequency varies from once a day to once a year. The duration of the attacks also varies greatly, from minutes to hours or even days. The attacks usually occur during the day; there is flaccid paralysis of the muscles of the limbs, especially of the proximal muscles of the legs. The reflexes are diminished or absent during an attack and it is frequently possible to elicit Chvostek's sign.

Attacks may be provoked by rest after intensive or prolonged muscular exercise, cold, fasting, and stress, but light muscular exercise or ingestion of carbohydrates (sugar cubes, bread) can have a favourable effect on an incipient attack. An attack can also be elicited by the oral administration of 4–5 g potassium chloride, preceded by intensive muscle exercise, if necessary. The serum potassium concentration is increased (5–7 mEq/l) during an attack as the potassium moves from the muscle to the blood. As a result there is also increased excretion of potassium in urine. The patient does not normally show any neurological abnormalities between attacks, although myotonia and sometimes weakness of the pelvic and shoulder girdle muscles may occur.

Glycogen-filled vacuoles are present in the muscle fibres during or immediately after the attack, and can be seen on muscle biopsy. Between attacks, tubular aggregates can be observed in type-II fibres. Since the attacks are rarely serious and do not last very long, therapy is not normally required during an attack. In the case of long-lasting and/or severe attacks, 1–2 g calcium gluconate can be given intravenously. An incipient attack can be terminated by 2–4 inhalations of salbutamol (200–400 mEq). Finally, attacks can be prevented by 250 mg acetazolamide 1–3 times a day.

23

Polymyositis and dermatomyositis

Polymyositis is a collective name for a group of non-hereditary and inflammatory myopathies. If the characteristic skin rash is present the term dermatomyositis is used. For that reason many authors prefer the term 'polymyositis–dermatomyositis complex' for this group of acquired diseases.

The cause of this condition is unknown. It is thought that

cellular and humoral immunologic mechanisms may play a role, especially since the condition sometimes occurs in collagen–vascular diseases (lupus erythematosus, panarteritis nodosa, rheumatoid arthritis, scleroderma) and because it responds well to treatment with corticosteroids and immunosuppressive drugs. Several classifications have been suggested (Table 23.1); as a rule they work well, although not always. In view of the similarity in clinical, electromyographical, histopathological and therapeutical aspects, for simplicity's sake it will be referred to below as 'the disease'. It is important to bear in mind though that 'the disease' in fact refers to a group of conditions.

Table 23.1. Classification of the polymyositis–dermatomyositis complex.

According to the Research Group on Neuromuscular Diseases of the World Federation of Neurology (1968).
(1) Polymyositis, acute, subacute or chronic.
(2) Polymyositis or dermatomyositis in collagen–vascular disease.
(3) Polymyositis or dermatomyositis in malignant disease.

According to Bohan and Peter (1975).
(1) Primary, idiopathic polymyositis.
(2) Primary, idiopathic dermatomyositis.
(3) Dermatomyositis (or polymyositis) associated with neoplasm.
(4) Childhood dermatomyositis (or polymyositis) associated with vasculitis.
(5) Polymyositis or dermatomyositis with associated collagen–vascular disease.

The disease is often observed in childhood (5–15 years, usually as dermatomyositis) and in middle-age (45–55 years). The onset may be acute and can lead to very severe muscle weakness within a few days. Signs of the disease are sometimes preceded by a general feeling of malaise. The muscles — especially those of the shoulder girdle and upper arms — can be painful and sensitive to pressure. More often though the disease will manifest as a gradual decrease in muscle power which can take from a couple of weeks to a few months. In this case there is no sense of malaise, fever, or muscle pain. The signs and symptoms suggest weakness of the muscles of the pelvic and shoulder girdles, and of the proximal musculature of the limbs. Weakness of the neck flexors also occurs frequently. Many patients complain of difficulty with swallowing and/or choking, while dysarthria (nasal speech) occurs relatively often. In the course of the disease the distal muscles may weaken. Polymyositis in which the muscle weakness is virtually limited to the distal muscles of the limbs has also been described. This is very rare however; the involvement of the extraocular and facial muscles is equally rare. Partially because of the relatively rapid onset of the muscle weakness there is no wasting, or very little, unless the disease shows a chronic course. It is also noteworthy that the reflexes are normal or slightly diminished, but never absent. Contractures may occur in chronic disease. The muscles may become calcified, especially if the patient is a child with acute polymyositis and dermatomyositis. It is possible to demonstrate the calcification by X-ray, for example, in the muscles of the upper arm and upper leg.

Patients with dermatomyositis typically have lilac erythematous facial eruption which extends butterfly-like over the nose, around the eyes, and across the cheeks and the forehead. The upper eyelids sometimes show marked dark-violet discoloration (heliotrope rash). In addition, a more or less scaly rash or telangiectasia can be observed on the neck, across the upper part of the chest (Fig. 23.1), on the extensor surfaces of the arms (Fig. 23.2) and upper legs, across the knuckles of the fingers, around the elbows, the knees and the medial malleoli. A hyperaemia caused by local vasculitis may occur around the finger nails. The skin and subcutaneous tissue may become oedematous in acute cases. Nodular calcifications and ulcerations may manifest in the more chronic cases.

Arthralgia is common, although it is usually mild, and does not last very long. In the case of severe joint complaints associated with swelling and redness, the possibility of a polymyositis associated with rheumatoid arthritis should be considered. Rheumatologists have pointed out that X-rays show dislocation or subluxation of the interphalangeal joint of the thumb. Raynaud's syndrome occurs in patients who also have a collagen disease. Interstitial pneumonitis and bronchiolitis, which may progress to fibrotic alveolitis at a later stage, probably occur more often than earlier assumed. The patients have a dry cough and minor effort is enough to make them short of breath. These signs are sometimes

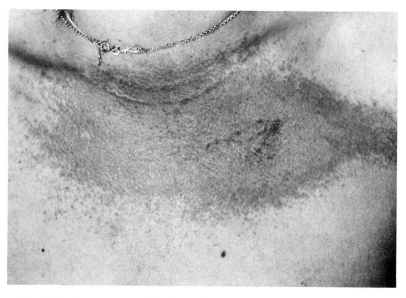

Fig. 23.1. Dermatomyositis. Extensive exanthema with typical location across the upper part of the chest.

seen to precede muscle weakness. Clinical cardiac signs are seen in only a minority of cases. In some series, however, the authors found arhythmias and conduction defects in the electrocardiogram of half the patients. Serum creatine kinase activity is almost always raised and can often rise to extremely high values (see Table 10.1, p. 69). There is no relationship between the severity of the muscle weakness and the concentration of serum creatine kinase. Serum myoglobin is also markedly increased, although myoglobinuria is rare (see Table 25.1, p. 145). The erythrocyte sedimentation rate is slightly increased in only half the patients, particularly in the acute cases.

The electromyogram may show abnormal spontaneous activity, including fibrillation potentials and positive sharp waves as well as bizarre high-frequency discharges. This is particularly evident in the paraspinal muscles. After voluntary contraction of the muscles one can usually observe brief polyphasic potentials with a low amplitude.

Apart from electromyography, serum myoglobulin and determining serum creatine kinase activity, muscle biopsy also makes an important contribution to the diagnosis. Structural changes (necrotic fibres, regenerating fibres), interstitial and perivascular cell infiltrates (mainly lymphocytes and plasma cells), and an increase in endomysial connective tissue are observed.

Atrophic fibres are sometimes seen on the edge of the fasciculi (perifascicular atrophy). An absence of cell infiltrates in the muscle biopsy does not exclude the presence of polymyositis. In this case, however, there should be other very strong arguments favouring this diagnosis (Table 23.2). On the other hand, the presence of cell infiltrates does not always indicate the existence of

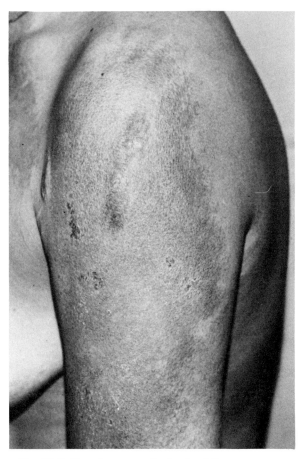

Fig. 23.2. Exanthema on the back of the upper arm.

Table 23.2 The polymyositis–dermatomyositis complex

Factors favouring the diagnosis.	*Factors possibly contradicting the diagnosis*
HISTORY	
Duration of complaints relatively short.	Hereditary occurrence.
Limb-girdle weakness.	Symptoms since birth or first year of life.
Dysphagia.	First signs in distal muscles.
Cutaneous manifestations.	Diplopia.
Muscular pain.	Muslce cramps.
Arthralgia.	Early appearance of contractures.
Raynaud's syndrome.	Fluctuation of signs.
Dyspnoea.	Signs and symptoms occurring in attacks.
Non-productive cough.	
NEUROLOGICAL EXAMINATION	
Limb-girdle syndrome.	Weakness of distal muscles.
Weakness of neck flexors.	Distal muscles more involved than proximal muscles.
Painful muscles.	
Painful joints.	Weakness of facial and/or extra-ocular muscles.
Slight muscular atrophy or none at all.	Marked atrophy of the muscles.
Tendon reflexes present.	Hypertrophy of calves.
	Tendon reflexes absent.
	Fasciculations.
	Myotonia.
GENERAL FINDINGS	
Collagen vascular disease.	Fever.
Neoplasia (in elderly patients).	Endocrine disorders.
Raynaud's syndrome.	
Dermatological features.	
LABORATORY FINDINGS	
Serum creatine kinase (very) high.	Serum creatine kinase normal.

Table 23.2 contd.

Factors favouring the diagnosis.	Factors possibly contradicting the diagnosis
Serum myoglobin (very) high.	Serum myoglobin normal.
EMG: spontaneous activity (paraspinal muscles.	EMG normal.
Nerve conduction velocities normal.	Nerve conduction velocities reduced.
Muscle biopsy: abundant structural changes, inflammatory cells, perifascicular atrophy.	Muscle biopsy: normal; neurogenic features; no inflammatory changes.
ECG: arthythmias; conduction defects.	
X-rays: chest (interstitial fibrosis) soft-tissue (calcifications); hands (arthritis, dislocation of interphalangeal thumb joints).	

polymyositis. Cell infiltrates can be a secondary sign in conditions associated with marked muscle fibre necrosis (as in rhabdomyolysis), but can also be seen in, for example, facioscapulohumeral dystrophy or amyotrophic lateral sclerosis. It is also important to bear in mind that a muscle biopsy from a part of a muscle which has been subject to EMG with needle electrodes or in which intramuscular injections were given, may show necrotic fibres and cell infiltrates ('needle myopathy').

Polymyositis and especially dermatomyositis are sometimes associated with malignant conditions such as carcinoma of the lung, breast, stomach, ovary, or uterus, or with sarcoma, leukemia, malignant lymphoma, and reticuloses. It is not known exactly how often such an association exists, and it varies in different series from 5 to 65 per cent. Some authors have suggested that it particularly affects men over the age of 40. This association does not occur in children with dermatomyositis. The signs of the polymyositis–dermatomyositis complex usually precede the signs of malignancy. For that reason many clinics will usually carry out an extensive investigation for the presence of an occult neoplasm in adults with polymyositis or dermatomyositis.

The treatment of choice for the polymyositis-dermatomyositis complex is, in the first instance, prednisone. The recommended dose is a single administration of 100 mg prednisone per day for a period of 4–8 weeks. After that the dose can be reduced gradually, for example, by giving 2.5 mg less every other day (100 mg–97.5 mg; 100 mg–95 mg; 100 mg–92.5 mg, etc.). Eventually, therefore, the patient will only be getting 100 mg prednisone, administered every other day. This should be kept up for 3 to 6 months, after which this dose also can be reduced (e.g. by 2.5 mg every 2 to 4 weeks). Often prednisone is first administered in too low a dose, and is then reduced too quickly (after 1 or 2 weeks). Moreover, the raised serum creatine kinase is more likely to be treated than the weakness of the patient. The lowering of serum creatine kinase activity by prednisone is an aspecific phenomenon which is also observed, for example, on giving prednisone to children with Duchenne muscular dystrophy.

It usually takes one or two months before muscle power improves in patients with polymyositis in whom serum creatine kinase activity has decreased as a result of the prednisone treatment. It is inadequate to reduce the prednisone dosage because of a reduction or normalization in serum creatine kinase. The decision whether to maintain or reduce a certain dosage of prednisone should only be based on clinical phenomena, (i.e. muscle power). If one is guided too much by serum creatine kinase concentrations, there is a tendency to increase the dose every time the concentration increases. Although clinical deterioration may be preceded by an increase in serum creatine kinase, we also know that many patients show marked fluctuations in enzyme activity during treatment with prednisone. On the other hand, it is possible gradually to lower the dose in patients who no longer show any weakness, although their serum creatine kinase activity is still high. Treatment with prednisone may have all kinds of adverse side-effects. Side-effects also occur if the drug is suddenly discontinued or the dosage is reduced too fast. For that reason long-term therapy of the polymyositis–dermatomyositis complex should only be carried out by experienced specialists. In so-called prednisone-resistant cases other immunosuppressive drugs may be given, especially azathioprine. Plasma exchange and total body irradiation can be considered for patients with serious weakness who do not respond to drugs.

A patient with polymyositis or dermatomyositis should be mobilized as soon as possible. During the very long period of drug therapy, physiotherapy is also required, mainly to prevent contractures. Not enough is known about therapy with muscle-strengthening exercises, though the general tendency seems to be one of reluctance to prescribe active exercise therapy.

Postscript

In every middle-aged patient who develops a limb-girdle syndrome within a period of several weeks or months without having a hereditary disease in the family, one should first think of polymyositis.

Polymyositis does not have to be associated with pain in the muscles.

Polymyositis does not have to be associated with an increased erythrocyte sedimentation rate.

Skin alterations may occur and disappear again before the muscle weakness becomes manifest.

When a diagnosis of polymyositis is strongly suspected, there is no harm in starting prednisone therapy before the results of the muscle biopsy are available.

Polymyositis is a disease which can be treated and cured. After prednisone treatment the patient is grateful for the disappearance of his muscle weakness.

So far not a single patient with muscle weakness has expressed gratitude because his creatine kinase activity returned to normal after prednisone treatment.

A patient with polymyositis with too low a dose of prednisone is being given short measure.

24

Neuromuscular disorders associated with endocrine diseases

Many endocrine diseases can be associated with muscle weakness (Table 24.1). Some authors then speak of endocrine myopathies, although in many cases electrophysiology and histopathology both show signs of a neuropathy.

In hyperthyroidism there is progressive external ophthalmoplegia associated with exophthalmus. Upward gaze is often affected first. This does not appear to be caused by weakness of the m.rectus superior but rather by fibrosis of the m.rectus inferior. The same holds for the often greatly limited abduction of the eyes which is caused by fibrosis of the m.rectus medialis. Ptosis and chemosis and, in serious cases, ulcers of the cornea and visual impairment may also occur.

The first symptoms of the disease may manifest before, during or after the occurrence of thyrotoxicosis, while a deterioration of the exophthalmus may occur in spite of successful treatment of the hyperthyroidism. Neuropathy of the optic nerve may also develop in this euthyroid phase.

Thyrotoxicosis may be associated with a chronic limb-girdle syndrome in which the weakness of the shoulder-girdle muscles is more marked than that of the pelvic-girdle muscles. In such cases marked atrophy of the muscles is sometimes seen too. The reflexes are usually brisk. Serum creatine kinase activity is usually normal. The electromyograph reveals brief low-voltage polyphasic action potentials. The muscle weakness, the atrophy, and the EMG abnormalities recover completely after treatment of the hyperthyroidism.

The association of hyperthyroidism with myasthenia gravis (in about 5 per cent of patients) and with hypokalaemic periodic paralysis (especially in Asians) is a phenomenon which is only partially understood.

Hypothyroidism may also be associated with muscle weakness (myxoedema-myopathy) which may be accompanied by muscle

Table 24.1 Neuromuscular syndromes in endocrine diseases.

Hyperthyroidism.	*Hypothyroidism.*
Ophthalmoplegia.	Myxoedema–myopathy.
Limb-girdle syndrome.	Kocher–Debré–Sémélaigne syndrome.
Polyneuropathy.	Hoffmann syndrome.
	Polyneuropathy.
	Carpal-tunnel syndrome.
Hyperparathyroidism.	
Limb-girdle syndrome.	
Acromegaly.	*Cushing syndrome.*
Limb-girdle syndrome.	Limb-girdle syndrome.
Polyneuropathy.	Polyneuropathy.
Carpal-tunnel syndrome.	
Addison's disease.	*Diabetes mellitus.*
Generalized muscle weakness.	Polyneuropathy.
Hyperkalaemic periodic paralysis.	Mononeuropathy.
	Multiple mononeuropathies.
	Radioculopathy.
Primary hyperaldosteronism.	
Hypokalaemic periodic paralysis.	
Limb-girdle syndrome.	

pains, cramps, and sometimes muscle hypertrophy. The reflexes, especially the ankle jerks, show a delayed relaxation. A ridge (myoedema), in the past mistaken for myotonia, may sometimes develop after percussion of the muscle with a percussion hammer. This phenomenon is not typical of hypothyroid myopathy; it can also be observed in cachectic patients. During the myoedema — which can sometimes last for one minute — there is no electrical activity and this also makes it different from myotonia. Serum creatine kinase activity is sometimes raised. In children with hypothyroidism, a marked hypertrophy of the muscles (Kocher–Debré–Sémélaigne syndrome) may occur in addition to muscle weakness. Painful muscle spasms and abnormally slow contraction and relaxation of the muscles may sometimes develop in adults with myxoedema and muscle hypertrophy (Hoffmann syndrome). A polyneuropathy with symptoms of both motor and sensory disorders may also occur. In addition, there may occur a compression, usually bilateral, of the median nerve in the carpal tunnel.

A proximal muscle weakness which is normally more marked in the lower limbs may develop in primary and secondary hyperparathyroidism. The muscles are often painful after exercise. Osteomalacia may cause so much pain in the bones that the testing of muscle function becomes very difficult. A severe weakness appears to exist but in reality the patient does not dare to move his limbs because of the pain this produces. The reflexes are usually very brisk. Serum creatine kinase activity is normal. The alkaline phosphatase concentration is usually increased, while in primary hyperparathyroidism, calcium is also raised. Surgery (removal of the adenoma) can be considered in primary hyperparathyroidism. Vitamin D (1,25-dihydroxy-calciferol; calcitriol) is given in osteomalacia. A complete recovery occurs in both cases.

25

Paroxysmal myoglobinuria

Myoglobin is a haem-containing globular protein which only occurs in the skeletal and cardiac muscle. When there is marked necrosis of muscle tissue, the blood myoglobin concentration is especially high. Myoglobin is excreted by the kidneys and causes the urine to turn a dark- to reddish-brown colour (myoglobinuria). There is no correlation between the myoglobin level in blood and the occurrence of myoglobinuria. The most sensitive method for demonstrating myoglobin in blood and urine is radio-immunoassay.

Myoglobinuria is a sign, not a disease. Only if no single cause of myoglobinuria can be found does one speak of idiopathic paroxysmal and paralytic myoglobinuria (Meyer–Betz disease). As myoglobinuria is often the result of a primary destruction of muscle fibres, some authors prefer the name rhabdomyolysis.

Attacks of myoglobinuria may be accompanied by general malaise, fever, nausea, vomiting, headache, and muscle pain. Apart from these, transient muscle weakness may also occur, especially in the muscles of the limbs. Sometimes myoglobinuria develops 2 to 24 hours after the muscle phenomena. Usually it is accompanied by a very large increase in serum creatine kinase activity. Myoglobinuria may be associated with numerous disorders (Table 25.1). Often there are several provoking factors, such as coma due to intoxication combined with arterial compression because the patient puts all his weight on his arm as he lies. Strenuous muscle exercise and heavy perspiration in hot weather, or fever with a status epilepticus are also combinations which may provoke myoglobinuria. A hazardous complication of myoglobinuria is tubular necrosis with acute renal failure.

Table 25.1. Diseases in which myoglobinuria may occur.

Muscle diseases.
Phosphorylase deficiency (McArdle's disease).
Phosphofructokinase deficiency.
Phosphoglycerate kinase deficiency.
Phosphoglycerate mutase deficiency.
Lactate dehydrogenase deficiency (M-subunit).
Carnitine palmityltransferase deficiency.
Polymyositis–dermatomyositis complex.
Malignant hyperthermia.

Excessive muscle use.
Military drill.
Marathon runners, skaters.
Status epilepticus.
Delirium tremens.
Myoclonia.

Muscle trauma.
Compression by heavy objects (crush injuries).
Compression by weight of own body (coma).

Table 25.2 (*cont.*)

Ischaemic muscle necrosis.
Arterial occlusion (thrombosis, embolism).
Arterial compression by trauma (see above).

Intoxication.
Alcohol.
Heroin.
Amphetamine.
Barbiturates.
Tranquillizers.
Cytostatics.
Carbon monoxide.
Clofibrate.
Succinylcholine.

Infectious diseases.
Tetanus.
Typhoid.
Herpes simplex.
Coxsackie infections.
Mononucleosis.
Influenza.

Hypokalaemia.
Gastrointestinal disorders.
Laxatives.
Diuretics.
Liquorice (glycyrrhizic acid).
Carbenoloxone sodium.

Idiopathic.
Paroxysmal, paralytic myoglobinuria or Meyer–Betz disease, sometimes
familial.

26

Malignant hyperthermia

Malignant hyperthermia, or malignant hyperpyrexia, is a syndrome with, as a rule, an autosomal dominant mode of inheritance and varying penetration. In patients at risk, the syndrome will develop during anaesthesia, especially with succinylcholine and halothane, although, in principle, many other muscle relaxants and anaesthetics may trigger off the condition.

At the beginning of anaesthesia, it appears impossible to obtain sufficient muscle relaxation in the patient, and at the same time the tone of the mm.masseteres increases. As a result the anaesthetist will experience difficulties with intubation and decide to increase (!) the dosage of the muscle relaxant and/or anaesthetic. This causes tachycardia and a strong generalized rigidity of the musculature. The rigidity may be absent in about a quarter of the patients (non-rigid form). Soon afterwards there will be a rapid and fulminating rise in body temperature, sometimes to above 40°C within 15 minutes. Severe respiratory and metabolic acidosis and hyperkalaemia develop with a possibility of the tachycardia eventually leading to ventricular fibrillation and death. If, however, the patient survives this serious condition very high serum creatine kinase activity is observed, as well as myoglobinuria.

To recognize a patient at risk, one should first take a very careful family history. Some high-risk patients may show alterations such as (aspecific) changes in the muscle biopsy or a slight increase in serum creatine kinase activity. There is an increased risk in patients with central core disease (see p. 99) and with chondrodystrophic myotonia (Schwartz–Jampel syndrome, see p. 107). In general, however, patients with other muscular diseases — particularly those with myotonic dystrophy or Duchenne muscular dystrophy — are not at an increased risk of developing this syndrome. On the other hand, however, Duchenne muscular dystrophy patients can die from cardiac arrest when given halothane and succinylcholine. In some clinics techniques have been developed which identify possible sensitivity to halothane. They rely on the *in-vitro* testing of muscle tissue.

It is assumed that the syndrome is the result of an accumulation of calcium in the sarcoplasm of the muscle fibres. Treatment with drugs is therefore aimed at lowering sarcoplasmic calcium. Especially good results are sometimes obtained by the intravenous administration of dantrolene sodium. Apart from this, treatment consists of the immediate discontinuation of anaesthesia, cooling the body and combating the acidosis. Nevertheless, mortality from malignant hyperthermia appears to be high.

27

Complaints about the muscles

Muscle cramps

Every doctor is regularly confronted with complaints of painful transient contractions of (part of) a muscle or a muscle group after spontaneous or voluntary muscle contraction. Everybody knows the symptom of muscle cramp from personal experience. Ordinary or benign muscle cramps can occur in young healthy adults as well as in older people. An increased tendency to muscle cramp is observed during pregnancy. Such cramps may occur at night in bed, especially in the muscles of the calves with plantar flexion of the toes or the entire foot. However, cramps may also occur in a variety of other muscles, especially after a strong contraction in an already shortened muscle or during or after heavy physical exercise. The muscle knots and the hardness may persist for several seconds or minutes. After persistent severe muscle cramp or a series of cramps, the muscle may remain sensitive or painful for days. In this case a slight increase in serum creatine kinase activity is observed. Fasciculations may be present prior to the muscle cramp or they may be observed shortly after the cramp has disappeared.

The mechanism of ordinary muscle cramps is unknown. Electromyography during cramp reveals episodic high-frequency action potentials emanating from part of the muscle. This activity rapidly spreads to the rest of the muscle. Muscle cramp can normally be halted by passive stretching of the muscle concerned. Benign nocturnal cramps can be treated with 200 mg quinine sulphate or with 200 mg chloroquine before going to sleep. In cramps occurring mostly in the daytime one can try phenytoin (e.g. 100 mg 3 times a day) or carbamazepine (e.g. 200 mg 3 times a day). The treatment of benign muscle cramp is, nevertheless, often unrewarding. Fortunately though, most patients show spontaneous remission.

Muscle cramps may be the first sign of a neuromuscular disease, for example, Becker muscular dystrophy (see p. 73) or amyotrophic lateral sclerosis (see p. 33). Muscle cramps may also occur in lower motor neuron disorders (spinal muscular atrophy, polyneuropathies and root lesions). The rare myopathies with tubular aggregates and familial AMP deaminase deficiency are also often associated with muscle cramp.

Muscle cramp must be distinguished from contracture; in the latter the entire muscle contracts, usually after (ischaemic) muscular exercise, and the pain lasts many minutes. Electro-myography during the contracture does not reveal any electrical activity in the muscle concerned. Muscle contracture is often observed in myophosphorylase deficiency (McArdle's disease, see p. 123) and phosphofructokinase deficiency (see p. 125). Muscle cramps should also be differentiated from spasms; these are also associated with painful contractions of muscles or muscle groups. Muscle spasms occur in central nervous system disorders (e.g. in lesions of the pyramidal tract and in the stiff-man syndrome). Finally, tetanus and myotonia should also be distinguished from muscle cramps, although myotonia, in particular, is rarely experienced as painful by the patient.

Fasciculations

Fasciculations develop due to spontaneous contraction of a group of muscle fibres. These involuntary muscle contractions, of which the pathogenesis remains unknown, are clearly visible in muscles located just under the skin. One may attempt to provoke suspected fasciculations by getting the patient to contract the muscle involved several times, or by giving it several blows with a percussion hammer. Cold can also provoke fasciculations. Most healthy people have noticed fasciculations at some time, especially in the muscles of the calves or small muscles of the hand. Sometimes they are also accompanied by muscle cramps. It is impossible to find any clinical or electromyographic difference between these benign fasciculations and those which occur in anterior horn cell disorders (amyotrophic lateral sclerosis; spinal muscular atrophy), and sometimes in neuropathies and root lesions. Fasciculations in the tongue have been described in hyperparathyroidism. Furthermore, continuous fasciculations are seen with Isaacs' syndrome (continuous muscle fibre activity), accompanied by muscle stiffness, mainly distal muscle weakness, and excessive perspiration. These signs respond very well to phenytoin or carbamazepine.

Muscle pain

Muscle pain as the only symptom of an existing neuromuscular disease is extremely rare. Nevertheless there are a number of neuromuscular diseases in which complaints about muscle pain arise (Table 27.1). To compensate for the reduced functioning of severely weakened muscles, certain other muscles may well be used to an excessive degree. This excess load may also give rise to muscle pain.

Table 27.1. Neuromuscular diseases associated with muscle pain.

Neuralgic amyotrophy.
Neuropathies (diabetes, alcohol).
Polymyositis–dermatomyositis complex.
Myoglobinuria (rhabdomyolysis).
Carnitine palmityltransferase deficiency.
Myophosphorylase deficiency.
Phosphofructokinase deficiency.
Lambert–Eaton syndrome.
Myopathy in osteomalacia.
Hypothyroid myopathy.

Fatigue

Fatigue is an aspecific complaint which may occur in a variety of organic and non-organic diseases. If after extensive examination — usually by a specialist in general medicine — no abnormalities are found, then a neuromuscular disease is often considered as a possible cause. In this instance one usually thinks of myasthenia gravis, but a patient with this disease rarely complains of fatigue. Myasthenia gravis (see p. 56) is not characterized by fatigue but rather by a fluctuating muscle weakness which can be provoked by muscle effort and which will reduce or disappear after rest. Patients with Lambert–Eaton syndrome (see p. 63) on the other hand do complain of fatigue, especially in the legs.

Fatigue which develops more rapidly than normal after muscular exercise is a complaint that many patients with a neuromuscular disease have. It occurs predominantly at the beginning of the disease when the muscle weakness is slight and the patient hardly aware of it (as, for example in amyotrophic lateral sclerosis). Thus, the patient continues his normal daily workload, but with an impaired muscle system. This will cost him more effort and energy than before, and lead to fatigue. At a later stage in the disease, when the weakness is manifest, the patient will adapt to his handicap and the complaint will often disappear.

Fatigue is often an important complaint of patients with a myopathy associated with morphologically abnormal mitochondria (see p. 103). This complaint may precede the signs of myopathy by months or even years. Fatigue and reduced stamina after muscular exercise are complaints presented by those who suffer from certain types of glycogen storage diseases (see p. 120) and AMP deaminase deficiency, and by some patients with a myopathy with tubular aggregates.

High serum creatine kinase activity

Chronically high serum creatine kinase activity can be found in some people without there being any other objective signs of neuromuscular disease. This is often the case in young men whose jobs involve heavy physical labour or who are active sportsmen. In them the serum creatine kinase activity is, on average, increased three- or fourfold. This finding is sometimes discovered by accident, at other times because of the patient's vague, aspecific muscle complaints (cramps, pains, feeling of fatigue) which prompt investigation.

Some people show a particular rise in serum creatine kinase activity (enzyme lability) after generalized or more localized (arms) exercise. There is no correlation between the level of serum creatine kinase activity and the duration or intensity of the muscular exercise which has preceded it. In these cases creatine kinase activity generally does not increase for 18–48 hours after exercise. Determination of the creatine kinase activity after a few days of very little physical exercise will reveal normal values and may well avoid unnecessary examination.

Furthermore, with raised serum creatine kinase activity, the patient should always be asked about the administration of intramuscular injections just before the examination. An extensive electromyographical examination can also give rise to a temporary increase in creatine kinase activity.

Additionally, one should exclude conditions such as AMP deaminase deficiency, hypothyroidism or hypoparathyroidism. The patient may also be susceptible to malignant hyperthermia, especially if he comes from a family with this syndrome. Women with raised creatine kinase activity can in theory be carriers of the gene for Duchenne muscular dystrophy or Becker muscular dystrophy.

Finally, there remain a number of patients whose chronically high serum creatine kinase activity remains totally unexplained. This is sometimes called idiopathic hyperCKaemia.

Bibliography

For more information the following books should be consulted:

Bethlem, J. (1980). *Myopathies.* 2nd edn. Elsevier North-Holland Biomedical Press, Amsterdam.

Brooke, M. H. (1986). *A clinician's view of neuromuscular diseases.* 2nd edn. The Williams & Wilkins Company, Baltimore.

Carpenter, S. and Karpati, G. (1984). *Pathology of skeletal muscle.* Churchill Livingstone, New York.

Dubowitz, V. (1980). *The floppy infant.* 2nd edn. William Heinemann Medical Books Ltd., London.

Dubowitz, V. (1985). *Muscle biopsy: a practical approach.* 2nd edn. Baillière Tindall, London.

Dijck, P. J., Thomas, P. K., Lambert, E. H. and Bunge, R. (1984). *Peripheral neuropathy.* Vol. 1 and 2. 2nd edn. W. B. Saunders Company, Philadelphia.

Engel, A. G. and Banker, B. Q. (eds.) (1986). *Myology. Basic and clinical.* McGraw-Hill, New York.

Goldensohn, E. S. and Appel, S. H. (ed.), (1977). *Scientific approaches to clinical neurology.* Vol. 2. Lea & Febiger, Philadelphia.

Harper, P. S. (1979). *Myotonic dystrophy.* W. B. Saunders Company, Philadelphia.

Kendall, H. O., Kendall, F. P. and Wadsworth, G. E. (1971). *Muscles. Testing and function.* 2nd edn. The Williams & Wilkins Company, Baltimore.

Layzer, R. B. (1985). *Neuromuscular manifestations of systemic disease.* F. A. Davis Company, Philadelphia.

Mulder, D. W. (1980). *The diagnosis and treatment of amyotrophic lateral sclerosis.* Houghton Mifflin Professional Publishers, Medical Division, Boston.

Oosterhuis, H. J. G. H. (1984). *Myasthenia gravis.* Churchill Livingstone, Edinburgh.

Pact, V., Sirotkin-Roses and Beatus, J. (1984). *The muscle testing handbook.* Little, Brown and Company, Boston.

Vinken, P. J. and Bruyn, G. W. (ed.) (1979). *Handbook of clinical neurology.* Vols 21, 22, 40 and 41. Elsevier North-Holland Publishing Company, Amsterdam.

Walton, J. N. (ed.) (1981). *Disorders of voluntary muscle.* 4th edn. Churchill Livingstone, Edinburgh.

153

Index